Endoscopy and Endosurgery

Guest Editor

STEPHEN J. DIVERS, BVetMed, DZooMed, DACZM, DipECZM(herp), FRCVS

VETERINARY CLINICS OF NORTH AMERICA: EXOTIC ANIMAL PRACTICE

www.vetexotic.theclinics.com

Consulting Editor
AGNES E. RUPLEY, DVM, Dipl. ABVP–Avian

May 2010 • Volume 13 • Number 2

SAUNDERS an imprint of ELSEVIER, Inc.

W.B. SAUNDERS COMPANY
A Division of Elsevier Inc.

1600 John F. Kennedy Boulevard • Suite 1800 • Philadelphia, Pennsylvania 19103-2899

http://www.vetexotic.theclinics.com

VETERINARY CLINICS OF NORTH AMERICA: EXOTIC ANIMAL PRACTICE Volume 13, Number 2
May 2010 ISSN 1094-9194, ISBN-13: 978-1-4377-1884-3

Editor: John Vassallo; j.vassallo@elsevier.com

Veterinary Clinics of North America: Exotic Animal Practice (ISSN 1094-9194) is published in January, May, and September by Elsevier, Inc., 360 Park Avenue South, New York, NY 10010-1710. Subscription prices are $198.00 per year for US individuals, $329.00 per year for US institutions, $103.00 per year for US students and residents, $234.00 per year for Canadian individuals, $388.00 per year for Canadian institutions, $264.00 per year for international individuals, $388.00 per year for international institutions and $132.00 per year for Canadian and foreign students/residents. To receive student/resident rate, orders must be accompanied by name of affiliated institution, date of term, and the *signature* of program/residency coordinator on institution letterhead. Orders will be billed at individual rate until proof of status is received. Foreign air speed delivery is included in all *Clinics* subscription prices. All prices are subject to change without notice. **POSTMASTER:** Send address changes to *Veterinary Clinics of North America: Exotic Animal Practice*, Elsevier Health Sciences Division, Subscription Customer Service, 3251 Riverport Lane, Maryland Heights, MO 63043. **Customer Service: Telephone: 1-800-654-2452** (U.S. and Canada); **1-314-447-8871** (outside U.S. and Canada). **Fax: 1-314-447-8029. E-mail: journalscustomerservice-usa@elsevier.com** (for print support); **journalsonlinesupport-usa@elsevier.com** (for online support).

Reprints. For copies of 100 or more of articles in this publication, please contact the Commercial Reprints Department, Elsevier Inc., 360 Park Avenue South, New York, New York 10010-1710. Tel.: (212)-633-3813; Fax: (212)-633-1935; E-mail: reprints@elsevier.com.

Veterinary Clinics of North America: Exotic Animal Practice is covered in *MEDLINE/PubMed (Index Medicus).*

Printed and bound in the United Kingdom

Transferred to Digital Print 2011

Contributors

CONSULTING EDITOR

AGNES E. RUPLEY, DVM
Diplomate, American Board of Veterinary Practitioners — Avian Practice; and Director and Chief Veterinarian, All Pets Medical and Laser Surgical Center, College Station, Texas

GUEST EDITOR

STEPHEN J. DIVERS, BVetMed, DZooMed, FRCVS
Diplomate, American College of Zoological Medicine; Diplomate, European College of Zoological Medicine (herpetology); Royal College of Veterinary Surgeons Recognized Specialist in Zoo and Wildlife Medicine, European Veterinary Specialist in Zoological Medicine (herpetology); Professor of Zoological Medicine, Department of Small Animal Medicine and Surgery, College of Veterinary Medicine, University of Georgia, Athens, Georgia

AUTHORS

STEPHEN J. DIVERS, BVetMed, DZooMed, FRCVS
Diplomate, American College of Zoological Medicine; Diplomate, European College of Zoological Medicine (herpetology); Royal College of Veterinary Surgeons Recognized Specialist in Zoo and Wildlife Medicine, European Veterinary Specialist in Zoological Medicine (herpetology); Professor of Zoological Medicine, Department of Small Animal Medicine and Surgery, College of Veterinary Medicine, University of Georgia, Athens, Georgia

CHARLES J. INNIS, VMD
Director, Animal Health Department, New England Aquarium, Central Wharf Boston, Massachusetts

DAN H. JOHNSON, DVM
Avian and Exotic Animal Care, Raleigh, North Carolina

MICHAEL J. MURRAY, DVM
Staff Veterinarian, Monterey Bay Aquarium, Monterey, California

MARK D. STETTER, DVM
Diplomate, American College of Zoological Medicine; Director, Department of Animal Health, Disney's Animal Programs, Lake Buena Vista, Florida

Contents

> The first descriptions of endoscopy date back to the times of Hippocrates
> (460–377 BC), who described the use of a rectal speculum in humans. Since
> that time, technologic advances have fueled the development of
> endoscopy equipment. The application of human pediatric instruments
> in exotic pet medicine has enabled these minimally invasive techniques
> to be applied to birds, reptiles, amphibians, fish, and small mammals.
> This article aims to summarize the development of endoscopy equipment
> and focuses on recent developments in miniature laparoscopy equipment
> that have found use in zoologic companion animal practice.

> Unlike most animals, birds are blessed by an air sac system that essentially
> provides the endoscopist with a preinsufflated patient. Thanks to this unique
> anatomy and the pioneering work of Greg Harrison, Michael Taylor, and
> other avian veterinarians, rigid endoscopy has enjoyed considerable popu-
> larity in avian practice over the past 30 years. Indeed, endoscopy now is
> considered an essential component of the avian investigation for many clin-
> ical presentations, and indeed few could argue that high-quality avian med-
> icine is possible without rigid endoscopy. The ability to examine the internal
> viscera, respiratory, gastrointestinal, and reproductive tracts, and collect
> samples for definitive diagnosis continues to play a central role in avian prac-
> tice, and this article summarizes the most common diagnostic endoscopic
> approaches likely to be undertaken in companion species.

> Endoscopy has proven to be an important diagnostic tool for avian veter-
> inarians wishing to visualize and biopsy internal structures. To date, most
> of the described endoscopic procedures are single-entry techniques. The
> use of miniature laparoscopy equipment has been pioneered in human pe-
> diatrics and many of these instruments now can be used used in zoologic
> companion animal practice. The addition of a second and third port using
> 2.5 or 3.5 mm cannulae has facilitated the use of 2 or 3 mm instruments
> within the avian coelom. Triangulation of various instruments, coupled
> with radiosurgical hemostasis, has made several procedures including
> salpingohysterectomy and orchidectomy possible endoscopically. In

addition, endoscope-assisted minimally invasive procedures including enterotomy, enterectomy, cloacopexy, and pneumotomy may be initiated internally and completed using more established techniques externally. The advent of minimally invasive endoscopic surgery offers significant benefits including rapid and accurate diagnosis, reduced need for an extensive coeliotomy, reduced surgical stress, more stable anesthesia, and reduced hospitalization periods.

The 2.7-mm telescope commonly used in avian practice has transitioned into an invaluable diagnostic tool for the reptile clinician. Previously plagued by vague medical histories, nonpathognomonic physical examinations, indistinct diagnostic images, and less than conclusive clinical pathology results, the reptile clinician often has had trouble making a definitive, antemortem diagnosis. A definitive diagnosis generally relies on the demonstration of a host pathologic response and the causative agent. The ability to examine internal structures and collect biopsies has enabled many postmortem diagnoses to now be appreciated in the living animal, and along with accurate diagnosis comes accurate prognosis and improved case management. The advent of 3-mm human pediatric laparoscopy equipment has fueled interest in minimally invasive endosurgery in exotic pets, including reptiles. However, the chelonian shell has also served as a catalyst to speed the development of surgical approaches to the coelom that do not involve major shell surgery. This article summarizes the most common endoscopic approaches in lizards, chelonians, and snakes for the purposes of making a diagnosis and increasingly performing endosurgery.

The development of endosurgical techniques for chelonians has reduced the need for more invasive approaches such as plastron osteotomy. Surgical access and manipulation of much of the coelomic viscera of chelonians can be accomplished using endoscopy. Endoscopic methods may be used to perform many chelonian reproductive surgical procedures, including oophorectomy, salpingotomy, salpingectomy, gender identification, and removal of ectopic eggs.

Despite the extensive use of endoscopy in avian and domestic animal practice, inclusion of exotic mammals (rabbits, rodents, ferrets, and so forth) in the endoscopist's case load is a much more recent phenomenon. Initially used as a means for the detailed evaluation of the oral cavity, rigid endoscopy has also become invaluable for the evaluation of the nasal cavity, urogenital tract, and increasingly for laparoscopic procedures. This article summarizes the most common procedures used by the author for first opinion and referral cases, and introduces some of the recent developments that are expected to become the standard of care in exotic animal practice in the future.

Rabbits, guinea pigs, chinchillas and many other small exotic mammals are not intubated routinely, because intubation requires specialized equipment and is difficult to perfect. Using a face mask for these species solely on the basis that they are unable to regurgitate ignores the numerous other benefits of airway control. This article summarizes the many advantages of endotracheal intubation and the various methods of intubation that have been reported. It introduces endoscopic intubation as a method that overcomes many of the difficulties associated with other methods and describes the equipment needed, how to intubate with an endoscope, how to confirm proper endotracheal tube placement, and possible complications. Over-the-endoscope intubation is discussed in detail, as it appears to provide the most versatile and reliable method of intubating exotic companion mammals.

Rigid laparoscopic surgery can be performed on bony fish. It is expected that laparoscopy will become a standard technique in veterinary medicine and will provide the zoo and aquarium clinician with a greater variety of diagnostic and therapeutic options. Laparoscopy has been found to be a very effective technique to directly visualize visceral organs and collect tissue samples. Although fish have significantly different anatomy as compared with terrestrial animals, the same laparoscopic principles can be applied successfully to this large and varied group of animals.

The importance of the shark species as ambassadors for the ocean ecosystems within public aquariums, and an ever increasing understanding of their importance as keystone species in those ecosystems, has resulted in more and more opportunities for the veterinary profession to interact with these charismatic fish. Although still in its infancy in aquatic medicine, endoscopy has the potential to be a valuable tool in the management of captive and free-ranging sharks. When contemplating an endoscopic procedure in a shark, the clinician must consider the unique anatomy of the species, the nature of the immobilization planned, and the performance of the procedure itself. Endoscopy should be considered as an adjunct procedure in the clinical management of captive sharks, and may have an important role in the scientific monitoring of free-ranging shark populations.

RELATED INTEREST

Veterinary Clinics of North America: Small Animal Practice
(Volume 39, Issue 5, September 2009)
Endoscopy
MaryAnn G. Radlinsky, DVM, MS, *Guest Editor*

THE CLINICS ARE NOW AVAILABLE ONLINE!

Access your subscription at:
www.theclinics.com

Preface

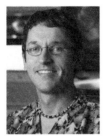

Stephen J. Divers, BVetMed, DZooMed, DACZM, DipECZM(herp), FRCVS
Guest Editor

My interest in endoscopy started as a veterinary student at the Royal Veterinary College, where, during various student externships, I was fortunate to be trained by private practitioners who taught me the benefits of minimally invasive techniques in zoological animals, particularly exotic pets. Soon after graduation in 1994, I traveled to the North American Veterinary Conference, where I undertook a 2-day course under the guidance of Drs Michael Taylor and Don Harris. The experience I gained there was the inciting cause for my subsequent career in endoscopy. Indeed, I was so impressed by the system and its ability to view with such clarity and collect biopsies inside a 400 gram pigeon that I immediately called my employer in England and asked for $12,000 for a basic endoscopy system. From his laughter at the end of the transatlantic phone line I detected that he was not going to provide me with the practice's credit card details! So I did what any foolish new graduate would do—I bought the system with my own money and traveled back to England, the proud owner of a new 2.7-mm system. In practice I was able to improve my skills on birds, reptiles, mammals, and fish. My employer at Elands Veterinary Clinic in Sevenoaks Kent, Dr Philip Lhermette, soon realized his error, and he too came to appreciate the true value of endoscopy in practice. Indeed, he later purchased my equipment and bought a load more. He went on to develop one of the most successful endoscopy referral centers in the United Kingdom and edited the recently published *British Small Animal Veterinary Association's Manual of Canine and Feline Endoscopy*. In 2001, I moved to the University of Georgia (UGA) to become a faculty member within the zoological medicine service. I was particularly fortunate to join the University at a time when Karl Storz Endoscopy was interested in UGA becoming their premier endoscopy training facility on the East Coast. After the installation of considerable equipment, combined with research facilities, and financial resources, I was able to undertake laboratory research and clinical studies to objectively assess the value of rigid endoscopy in reptiles, birds, and fish. I was like a kid in a candy store, and was fortunate enough to get paid for doing what I really enjoyed! My collaborative efforts with Drs Heather Barron, Scott Stahl, Charles Innis, Jan Hoover,

Vet Clin Exot Anim 13 (2010) ix–x
doi:10.1016/j.cvex.2010.01.009
1094-9194/10/$ – see front matter

Jay Shelton, MaryAnn Radlinsky, Clarence Rawlings, Bran Ricthie, Sam Dover, Sam Rivera, and others have concentrated on technique and procedural development, lab animal studies to determine efficacy and safety, and clinical research into practical application.

As someone who is not on the payroll of any company, I feel free to mention without complaint the support that Karl Storz Endoscopy (especially Christopher Chamness, Doug Merker, and Mike Bateman) and Ellman Radiosurgery (especially Richard Noss) have given to the veterinary profession. If it were not for their unwavering support, many research projects would never have been possible, and most training opportunities would disappear. Indeed, the original Mr Karl Storz was a great supporter of veterinarians, and his company continues to support research, development, and training within the veterinary profession despite the limited financial returns compared to the human market.

I am humbly indebted to the following veterinarians, who have selflessly provided training, encouragement, and mentorship to me over the years. I have no doubt that I am standing upon their shoulders as I attempt to advance the practice of endoscopy within zoological medicine: Dermod Malley, Neil Forbes, Philip Lhermette, John Cooper, James Carpenter, Scott Stahl, Charles Innis, Michael Taylor, Michael Murray, Mark Stetter, Fredric Frye, Peer Zwart, Christopher Chamness, Heather Barron, and Clarence Rawlings. In addition, this issue would not have been possible without the dedication of several long-term friends and colleagues who found it difficult to say no to a request to share their knowledge and expertise. Charles "Chuckles" Innis has been a long-time friend and colleague within the *Association* of Reptilian and Amphibian Veterinarians and has extensive expertise in chelonian reproduction and endoscopy. Indeed, he will be collaborator on a project to develop an endoscopic castration technique for chelonians this summer. Dan Johnson is very active within the *Association of Exotic Mammal Veterinarians*, and as a practitioner dealing with many small exotic mammals his descriptions of endoscopic intubation should bring relief to many of us who struggle with these challenging animals. Mike 'The Murr' Murray and Mark Stetter are 2 of the top fish veterinarians in the United States (although they might never admit to it), and given the increasing interest in these animals, both in private practice and aquaria, their articles on bony fish and elasmobranch endoscopy are unique and practical.

While I hope that these color articles will fan the flame of desire to wield an endoscope, no amount of literature can replace hands-on training. Fortunately, 2010 promises to be a bumper year for courses, with 4 to 8 hour practical courses being offered at AAV, ARAV and AAZV conferences this year. In addition, the extensive 2-day exotic pet endoscopy course at UGA (Dec 11–12, 2010) concentrates on pet birds, reptiles and mammals, and provides 15 hours of instruction and practical time. Course information and registration details are available from melissak@uga.edu, http://www.vet.uga.edu/CE/calendar/index.php. Happy scoping!

Stephen J. Divers, BVetMed, DZooMed, DACZM, DipECZM(herp), FRCVS
Department of Small Animal Medicine and Surgery (Zoological Medicine)
College of Veterinary Medicine
University of Georgia, 501 DW Brooks Drive
Athens, GA 30602, USA

E-mail address:
sdivers@uga.edu

Endoscopy Equipment and Instrumentation for Use in Exotic Animal Medicine

Stephen J. Divers, BVetMed, DZooMed, DACZM, DipECZM(herp), FRCVS

KEYWORDS

- Endoscopy • Equipment • Instrumentation
- Minimally invasive surgery • Exotic animal medicine
- Zoological medicine

DEFINITIONS, HISTORY, AND DEVELOPMENT

The term *endoscopy* is derived from the Latin *endo*, meaning "inside," and *scopein*, meaning "to view." The ability to evaluate internal structures is not new, with the earliest reports by Hippocrates (460–377 BC), who described the use of a rectal speculum. The development of electrical circuits, lamps, and metal tubes with simple glass lenses allowed rigid endoscopy to progress throughout the nineteenth and early twentieth centuries. The development of the rod-lens telescope with fiberoptic light transmission by Hopkins (1965) and charged-couple devices and digital imaging by Bell Laboratories (1969) have enabled instrument miniaturization while maintaining high-quality imagery.[1]

There are more than 100 million exotic pets in the United States compared with approximately 70 million dogs and 80 million cats.[2] Unlike in domestic animal medicine, there are few serologic tests available, especially in avian and reptile medicine; therefore, a definitive diagnosis often relies on the demonstration of a host pathologic response (eg, by histopathology, cytology, or paired rising titers) and identification the causative agent (eg, by microbiology, parasitology, or toxicology). Because of the difficulties of achieving a definitive antemortem diagnosis, many exotic animal diseases have traditionally been identified ante-mortem at organ level (eg, avian liver disease or iguana renal disease). Endoscopy offers a minimally invasive means of collecting biopsies, hence achieving a definitive diagnosis, which in turns enables more accurate and targeted therapy and improved case success. Today, with cost-effective

Department of Small Animal Medicine and Surgery (Zoological Medicine), College of Veterinary Medicine, University of Georgia, 501 DW Brooks Drive, Athens, GA 30602, USA
E-mail address: sdivers@uga.edu

Vet Clin Exot Anim 13 (2010) 171–185
doi:10.1016/j.cvex.2010.01.001
1094-9194/10/$ – see front matter

Table 1
Endoscopic instrumentation for companion exotic mammals, reptiles, birds, and fish

Equipment Description	Primary Indications
Telescopes and Endoscopes	
1-mm × 20-cm semirigid miniscope, 0°	Stomatoscopy, otoscopy, rhinoscopy, and tracheoscopy in animals up to 1 kg
1.9-mm × 18.5-cm telescope, 30° oblique, with integrated 3.3-mm operating sheath	Stomatoscopy, otoscopy, rhinoscopy, tracheoscopy, gastroscopy, colonoscopy, cloacoscopy, and coelioscopy in animals up to 3–4 kg
2.7-mm × 18-cm telescope, 30° oblique 4.8-mm operating sheath	Stomatoscopy, otoscopy, rhinoscopy, tracheoscopy, gastroscopy, colonoscopy, cloacoscopy, and coelioscopy in animals between 100 g and 10 kg
5-mm × 8.5-cm otoendoscope, 0°, with integrated operating sheath	Stomatoscopy and otoscopy in animals between 1 and 50 kg
Visualization and documentation	
Endovideo camera and monitor Xenon light source and light guide cable Digital capture device (eg, AIDA DVD, Karl Storz)	Required for all endoscopy procedures
Flexible instruments for use with operating sheaths	
1-mm biopsy forceps 1-mm grasping forceps	For use with 1.9-mm telescope and integrated sheath
1.7-mm biopsy forceps 1.3-mm single-action scissors 1.7-mm remote injection needle 1.7-mm grasping/retrieval forceps 1.7-mm wire basket retrieval 1.7-mm needle end radiosurgery electrode 1.7-mm polypectomy snare	For use with 2.7-mm telescope and 4.8-mm operating sheath and 5-mm otoendoscope
Insufflation	
CO_2 insufflator with silicone tubing	Used for insufflation during reptile/mammal coelioscopy/laparoscopy
Sterile saline suspended above endoscopy table with intravenous drip line to a port on the operating sheath	Used for sterile saline infusion for otoscopy, rhinoscopy, cystoscopy, cloacoscopy, and reptile (especially of small or aquatic species) or fish coelioscopy.
Rigid instruments, handles, and cannulae for multiple-entry coelioscopy	
2.5-mm graphite and plastic cannula 2-mm Reddick-Olsen dissecting forceps, plastic handle without racket 2-mm Metzenbaum scissors, plastic handle without racket 2-mm Babcock forceps, plastic handle with racket	Used with the 1.9-mm telescope for coelioscopy in animals under 1 kg

(continued on next page)

Table 1
(continued)

Equipment Description	Primary Indications
3.9-mm graphite and plastic cannula (accommodates 2.7-mm telescope and 3.5-mm protection sheath)	Used with the 2.7-mm telescope for coelioscopy in animals under 10 kg
3.5-mm graphite and plastic cannula (accommodates 3-mm instruments)	
3-mm fenestrated grasping forceps	
3-mm Reddick-Olsen dissecting and grasping forceps	
3-mm short curved Kelly dissecting and grasping forceps	
3-mm atraumatic dissecting and grasping forceps	
3-mm Babcock forceps	
3-mm Blakesley dissecting and biopsy forceps	
3-mm scissors with serrated, curved, double-action jaws	
3-mm microhook scissors, single-action jaws	
3-mm Mahnes bipolar coagulation forceps	
3-mm irrigation and suction cannula	
3-mm palpation probe with centimeter markings	
3-mm distendable palpation probe	
3-mm ultramicroneedle holder	
3-mm knot tier for extracorporeal suturing	
2 plastic handles without rackets	
1 plastic handle with Mahnes-style racket	
1 plastic handle with hemostat-style racket	
Radiosurgery equipment	
3.8- or 4.0-MHz dual radiofrequency unit with foot pedal (Ellman International)	Enables endoscopic instruments to be used as monopolar devices and facilitates bipolar coagulation
Monopolar lead to connect to plastic instrument handles	
Bipolar lead to connect to 3-mm Mahnes bipolar coagulation forceps	

equipment commonly available, it is difficult for veterinarians to offer an appropriate standard of care for birds, reptiles, and fish without endoscopy.

Rigid endoscopy has proved a useful diagnostic tool in veterinary medicine. The major advantages of endoscopy over traditional methods are (1) the ability to clearly visualize internal structures with magnification, (2) the ability to collect samples and biopsies for laboratory analyses, and (3) an increasing ability to perform minimally invasive endosurgery.[3,4] In the field of zoologic medicine, the application of diagnostic endoscopy was first adopted by avian veterinarians but has subsequently gained acceptance in a wide variety of zoologic areas, including exotic pets.

INSTRUMENTATION AND GENERAL TECHNIQUE

Given the variation in size, species-specific anatomy, and procedures that may be performed, a selection of different endoscopes and instruments is recommended (**Table 1**). The 2.7-mm system is most widespread in zoological companion animal practice, offers greatest versatility, and can be expanded as individual practice case-load dictates.[5–7] This system offers several advantages including single-entry procedures, ports for gas or fluid infusion, and an operating channel for the introduction of 1.7-mm (5F) instruments (**Fig. 1**). In addition, the 1.9-mm telescope with integrated sheath and the 1-mm semirigid miniscope are extremely useful for smaller species (**Fig. 2**).

The telescope is connected via a fiberoptic light guide cable to a light source (**Fig. 3**). Although halogen light sources are cheaper and effective for small (<2 kg) animals, xenon light sources provide better-quality light and an intensity that can illuminate the body cavities of large animals. An endovideo camera connected to the eyepiece of the telescope, although once considered a luxury addition, is an integral part of the endoscopy system and greatly facilitates surgeon performance (**Fig. 4**). Cameras, available in European PAL (Phase Alternating Line) and American NTSC (National Television System Committee) formats, can vary dramatically in cost from budget single-chip cameras to 3-chip, digital, high-definition models. Any camera, however cheap, greatly improves performance compared with using an eyepiece, and facilitates photodocumentation. The Tele Pack system combines a hybrid xenon light source, endovideo camera, LCD (Liquid Crystal Display) monitor, and a PCMCIA (Personal Computer Memory Card International Association) card slot for digital image capture and storage into a portable unit that is well suited for veterinarians working in the field

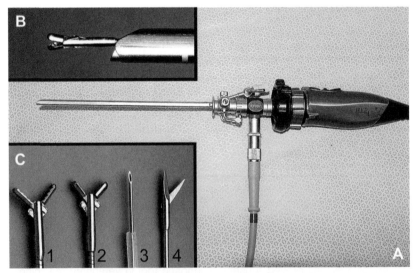

Fig. 1. A 2.7-mm telescope system (Karl Storz). (*A*) A 2.7-mm telescope housed within a 4.8-mm operating sheath, connected to a light cable and an endovideo camera. (*B*) A 1.7-mm biopsy forceps inserted down the instrument channel and emerging directly in front of the telescope. (*C*) A variety of instruments can be used through the operating channel, including 1.7-mm retrieval forceps (1), 1.7-mm biopsy forceps (2), remote injection/aspiration needle (3), and 1.3-mm single-action scissors (4). (*Courtesy of* Stephen J. Divers, Athens, GA.)

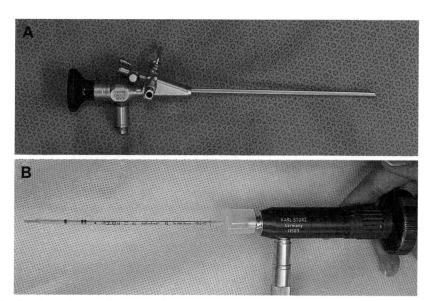

Fig. 2. (*A*) A 1.9-mm telescope with integrated operating sheath (Karl Storz). (*B*) A 1-mm semirigid miniscope (Karl Storz) with a 2-mm endotracheal tube placed over the endoscope in preparation for endotracheal intubation. (*Courtesy of* Stephen J. Divers, Athens, GA.)

(**Fig. 5**). Operating room setup is important and the monitor should be positioned directly in front of the endoscopist, with instruments within easy reach (**Fig. 6**).

Some form of insufflation is required for most coelioscopic/laparoscopic procedures (except in birds where the endoscope enters the air sac system). CO_2 gas delivered by a dedicated endoflator is preferred (**Fig. 7**), but air delivered by syringe or a small aquarium air pump can be used, as long as the risks associated with air emboli are not ignored. In some situations, the use of sterile saline infusion can be helpful, in particular when dealing with a hollow viscus (gastrointestinal tract, bladder, cloaca, etc), and is also preferred for aquatic animal coelioscopy because of the potential for residual insufflation gas to adversely affect postoperative buoyancy (**Fig. 8**).

The fact that most exotic pets weigh less than 2 kg requires careful control of the telescope with an eyepiece and camera supported using the superior hand and the

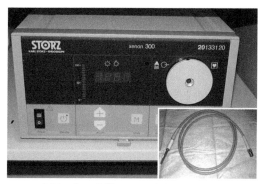

Fig. 3. Xenon light source (300 W) and fiberoptic light cable (Karl Storz) (*insert*). (*Courtesy of* Stephen J. Divers, Athens, GA.)

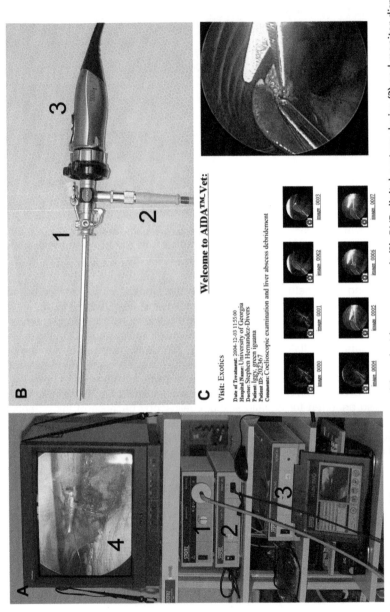

Fig. 4. (A) Rigid endoscopy tower with xenon light source (1), endovideo camera unit (2), DVD digital capture device (3) and monitor display (4) (Karl Storz). (B) Sheathed 2.7-mm telescope (1) attached to the light guide cable (2), and an Image-1 digital camera with zoom and digital interface functions (3) (Karl Storz). (C) Typical case photodocumentation obtained using an AIDA-Vet CD digital capture device (Karl Storz). (Courtesy of Stephen J. Divers, Athens, GA.)

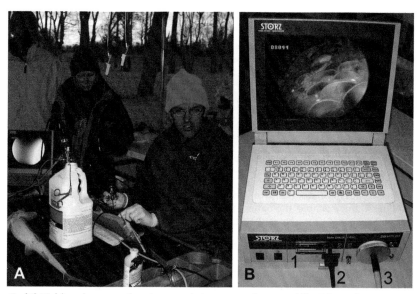

Fig. 5. (*A*) Field endoscopy of endangered sturgeon using a mobile Tele Pack system. These small compact units are well suited for mobile veterinary clinics or zoo and wildlife work. (*B*) Close-up of the Tele Pack (Karl Storz) demonstrating PCMCIA card for digital still capture (1), the camera unit (2), and light source (3). (*Courtesy of* Stephen J. Divers, Athens, GA.)

distal shaft of the telescope held by thumb and forefinger of the inferior hand (**Fig. 9**A). Handling the telescope in this fashion provides fine control without tremor.

Biopsies can be easily harvested from most structures. To insert and manipulate the instruments it is necessary to change from a 2-handed hold to a 1-handed technique. The usual thumb and forefinger support of the telescope shaft is adjusted so that the inferior hand takes the entire weight of the sheath-telescope-camera system. The

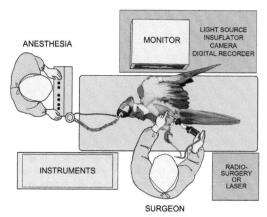

Fig. 6. Operating room setup is important and the monitor should be positioned directly in front of the endoscopist, with instruments within easy reach. (*Courtesy of* Stephen J. Divers, Athens, GA.)

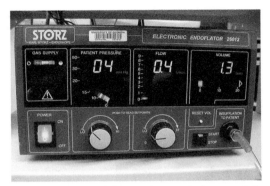

Fig. 7. Electronic endoflator (Karl Storz) designed to precisely control the delivery of CO_2 for insufflation. In this example, the patient pressure has been set to 4 mm Hg, with a CO_2 flow rate set to 0.4 L/min. So far a total of 1.3 L of CO_2 has been delivered. (*Courtesy of* Stephen J. Divers, Athens, GA.)

thumb is slid up the shaft of the sheath, and the fingers are curled over the top to encircle the sheath. When the sheath is grasped in a fist with the sheath further supported by the thumb to prevent rotation, the superior hand can be removed to pick up and insert an instrument down the operating channel (see **Fig. 9**B). This can only be performed using a correctly sheathed telescope; damage will otherwise occur.

The 1.0- and 1.7-mm (3F and 5F) grasping forceps are useful for manipulating tissues, débridement, and retrieving foreign objects or parasites. The fine-needle aspiration/injection can be used for the aspiration of fluid from cystic structures where biopsy may be contraindicated due to postsampling leakage. The needle can also be used for irrigation and drug administration. The 1.0- and 1.7-mm flexible biopsy forceps are used to harvest tissue samples for histopathology and microbiology in patients as small as 30 g. The small sample size usually permits collection of several biopsies for multiple laboratory tests and serial biopsies to monitor disease

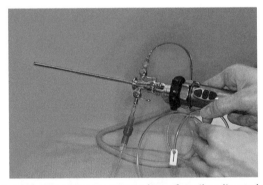

Fig. 8. A simple saline infusion system requires a bag of sterile saline to be suspended above the animal (not shown) and an ingress fluid delivery line attached to 1 of the ports on the 4.8-mm operating sheath (Karl Storz). A second delivery line is used as an egress and empties into a bucket under the table. By adjusting the sheath ports, an endoscopist can control the rate of fluid entering and leaving an area. Such a system works well for fish and turtle coelioscopy, avian and reptile cloacoscopy, and gastrointestinal evaluations. It is important that the temperature of the saline is similar to the patient's to avoid inducing hypothermia. (*Courtesy of* Stephen J. Divers, Athens, GA.)

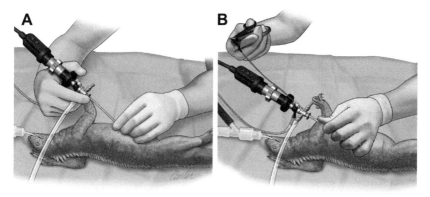

Fig. 9. Correct handling of the 2.7-mm telescope and 4.8-mm operating sheath. (*A*) The 2-handed technique for general evaluation involves supporting the sheathed telescope and camera with the superior hand while the thumb and forefinger of the inferior hand provide fine motor control without tremor. (*B*) The 1-handed technique facilitates instrument use by a single surgeon and involves the inferior hand taking the weight of the sheathed telescope and camera by gripping the entire shaft, with the thumb slid up the sheath to prevent rotation. The inferior hand is free to pick up and insert an instrument down the operating channel. (*Courtesy of* Stephen J. Divers, Athens, GA.)

progression over time to assess response to treatment. To take a tissue sample, the biopsy forceps are inserted down the operating channel and into the field of view (see **Fig. 1**B). It is easier to advance and manipulate the sheath-telescope-instrument as a single device than to try and keep the sheath-telescope still and independently move the biopsy forceps back and forth. With the biopsy forceps held open, the sheath-telescope-instrument is advanced to the tissue of interest and when tissue enters the biopsy cup, the jaws are gently closed. These instruments are delicate and the biopsy handle is only required to open the biopsy jaws. The handle's spring mechanism is usually sufficient to take a soft tissue biopsy without additional manual pressure, as long as the instrument is sharp. Clamping down on the handle damages the forceps and increases biopsy crush artifact. Some organs may be protected by a more fibrous membrane. The fixed blade of the 1.3-mm (4 Fr) scissors is inserted at a shallow angle through the membrane, and the sheath-telescope-scissors are advanced as a single unit, cutting the membrane as they proceed. The scissors can then be replaced by the biopsy forceps to take a sample through the capsular incision.

Biopsies are delicate and measure approx 2.5 mm^3 in size when collected using a 1.7-mm instrument. Handling and other histologic artifacts are reduced by gently dislodging the tissue from the biopsy cups into a small volume of sterile saline, before decanting into a biopsy cassette or bag and submitting in 10% neutral buffered formalin. Picking the biopsy out of the instrument using a needle causes severe damage, and even moistened cotton-tipped applicators can cause tissue alteration. Biopsies for microbiology are best submitted in sterile saline for immediate processing. Alternatively, if they are mailed to a laboratory, they should be submitted in appropriate transport media. For the submission of samples for toxicology or parasitology, it is wise to consult with the laboratory before sample collection.

A definitive diagnosis is important to maximize treatment success, and many exotic animal cases are unsuccessfully managed simply because of failure to identify the specific problem. Definitive diagnosis relies on the demonstration of a host pathologic response (by histopathology, less reliably by cytology, or using paired rising antibody titers) and the causative agent (by microbiology, parasitology, or toxicology). There are few reliable serologic tests available for most exotic species, and those that are available require a minimum of 2 to 3 weeks for endotherms and 6 to 9 weeks for ectotherms to demonstrate the necessary 2-fold increase in titers. It is, therefore, clear that tissue samples offer the most expedient means to a diagnosis, and endoscopy offers the least invasive antemortem method to collect such material. Consequently, clinicians have discovered that diagnostic endoscopy offers an unparalleled ability to facilitate antemortem diagnosis and maximize treatment success in many cases.

To evolve from purely diagnostic (observation and biopsy) to endosurgery, accurate hemostasis becomes increasingly critical. Radiosurgical and laser devices have become available to veterinarians and have facilitated the ability to incise and débride internally without significant hemorrhage. Diode lasers (AccuVet, Lumenis, Norwood, Massachusetts) are by design able to pass through flexible fiberoptic probes that can be inserted through instrument channels or cannulae (**Fig. 10**).[8,9] A variety of diode laser probes are available; however, 400- 600-μm conical or flat tips at 2 to 10 W are preferred (Surgimedics, The Woodlands, Texas). Until recently CO_2 lasers (AccuVet, Lumenis) could not be used via endoscopic instrument channels because of the inflexible nature of the ceramic delivery probes. The development of a long semirigid probe (AccuVet, Lumenis), however, has enabled the use of the CO_2 laser via the 1.7-mm instrument channel of the 4.8-mm operating sheath, but, although functional, it is unwieldy (**Fig. 11**). A variety of radiosurgery devices are available for use with foot-pedal activated 3.8- and 4.0-MHz radiosurgery units (Ellman International, Oceanside, New York) (**Fig. 12**), the most useful of which include various needle electrodes (Ellman International), bipolar forceps, and retractable polypectomy snare (Karl Storz Veterinary Endoscopy America). The degree of radiosurgical power required during endosurgery varies with operating conditions and the instrument used, but because of the microsurgical nature of most endosurgical procedures, lower settings are generally required compared with open surgery. Considerable growth in endoscopic radiosurgery has led to the availability of many monopolar and bipolar devices.

The recent availability of 2- and 3-mm human pediatric laparoscopy instruments (Karl Storz Veterinary Endoscopy America) has facilitated the development of

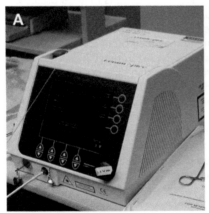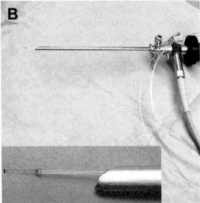

Fig. 10. (*A*) A 980-μm diode laser unit. (*B*) A 600-μm diode laser fiber inserted down the instrument channel of the 4.8-mm operating sheath, and emanating from the terminal end of the sheath in front of the terminal telescope lens (*insert*). (*Courtesy of* Stephen J. Divers, Athens, GA.)

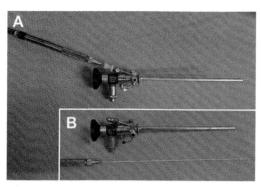

Fig. 11. (*A*) Elongated ceramic CO_2 laser tip inserted down the instrument channel of the 4.8-mm operating sheath. (*B*) The same ceramic tip alongside the sheath. (*Courtesy of* Stephen J. Divers, Athens, GA.)

multiple-entry endoscopy in small exotic species (**Fig. 13**).[10] Although the telescope is still used to provide visualization, additional operating cannulae provide access ports for the insertion of additional instruments. Instrument triangulation permits surgery without the need for extensive coeliotomy/laparotomy. Each additional access port is created using a 2.5- or 3.5-mm cannula. The cannulae are of surgical steel or graphite/plastic construction and have internal valves and optional insufflation stopcocks for gas delivery (**Fig. 14**). These valves are designed to prevent loss of CO_2 during insufflation. Although CO_2 insufflation is contraindicated when working within the avian air sac system, these valves are essential for preventing gas exchange between the respiratory system and the environment and, therefore, assist in maintaining safe and effective anesthesia. Insufflation stopcocks on cannulae are optional but are not required for avian coelioscopy and should be closed if present; however, they are essential when using the same system with mammals, reptiles, amphibians,

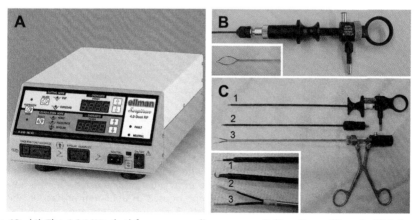

Fig. 12. (*A*) The 4.0-MHz dual frequency radiosurgery unit (Surgitron, Ellman). (*B*) Polypectomy snare hand-piece with extended end shown (*insert*) (Karl Storz). (*C*) Various radiosurgical endoscopic devices (Karl Storz): retractable needle (1), dissecting hook (2), and bipolar forceps (3). Close-up of instrument ends also shown (*insert*). (*Courtesy of* Stephen J. Divers, Athens, GA.)

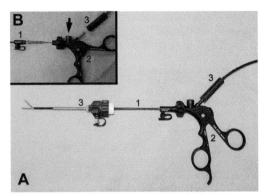

Fig. 13. Human pediatric 3-mm laparoscopy equipment (Karl Storz). (*A*) A 3-mm instrument (1) attached to a standard ClickLine handle (2). The instrument, attached to a radiosurgery unit via a connector on the handle (3), has been inserted through a 3.5-mm graphite/plastic cannula (3). (*B*) Instrument (1) and handle (2) can be quickly exchanged by pressing on the release button (*arrow*). The radiosurgical connection is also shown (3). (*Courtesy of* Stephen J. Divers, Athens, GA.)

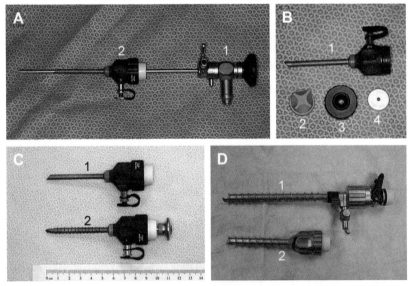

Fig. 14. Cannulae and trocars (Karl Storz). (*A*) A 2.7-mm telescope within a 3.5-mm protection sheath (1) inserted through a 3.9-mm × 10-cm graphite/plastic cannula with insufflation side port (2). (*B*) A 3.9-mm × 10-cm graphite/plastic cannula disassembled to illustrate the graphite cannula (1), leaflet valve (2), screw cap (3), and instrument seal (4). (*C*) A 3.9-mm × 10-cm graphite/plastic cannula with insufflation side port (1) and 3.5-mm × 10-cm threaded cannula with insufflation side port and trocar inserted (2). The 3.9-mm cannula can accommodate the 2.7-mm telescope housed in a 3.5-mm protection sheath whereas the 3.5-mm cannula can accommodate 3-mm instruments and, thanks to the threaded design, resists dislodgement in small exotic species. (*D*) Ternamian endotip cannulae: 6-mm × 15-cm cannula with insufflation side port and multifunctional valve (1) and 6-mm × 10.5-cm cannula with silicone leaflet valve. These metal cannulae are far heavier than the graphite/plastic type and best restricted to animals greater than 10 kg. (*Courtesy of* Stephen J. Divers, Athens, GA.)

or fish. The metal cannulae are more robust and heavier and, therefore, are used only for the larger animals. The plastic-graphite models are light and ideally suited to most exotic pet species.

The Ternamian endotip cannula is a recent improvement that has an external screw thread to enable gradual advancement by rotation (see **Fig. 14**C, D).[11] The cannula does not require trocar or axial penetration force during insertion. A telescope within the cannula provides a magnified view during entry. As the cannula is advanced, the fascia and the muscle fibers spread radially and are transposed onto the cannula's outer thread. The thin air sac (aves) or peritoneal membrane (non-aves) is transilluminated so that viscera, vessels, or adhesions are visualized before entry. The risks of iatrogenic visceral damage are therefore greatly reduced. A 3.9-mm graphite/plastic endotip cannula can be used with a 2.7-mm telescope sheathed within a 3.5-mm protection sheath (see **Fig. 14**A).

There are several size classes of instruments/cannulae, including 5 mm/6 mm, 3 mm/3.5 mm, and 2 mm/2.5 mm. Currently, 2-mm instruments are limited to Babcock forceps, dissecting forceps, and scissors. A greater variety of 3-mm instruments, however, are available, including dissection forceps, grasping forceps, scissors, biopsy forceps, palpation probes, and irrigation cannulae (**Fig. 15**). The largest variety of instruments can be found in 5-mm sizes due to their frequent use in human medicine. All these instruments have a standard attachment that enables them to be used

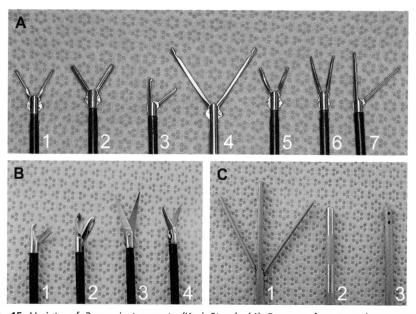

Fig. 15. Variety of 3-mm instruments (Karl Storz). (*A*) Forceps: fenestrated atraumatic grasping forceps (1), Reddick-Olsen dissecting forceps (2), small Babcock forceps (3), large Babcock forceps (4), short curved Kelly dissecting and grasping forceps (5), long curved Kelly dissecting and grasping forceps (6), and atraumatic dissecting and grasping forceps with single-action jaws (7). (*B*) Scissors and biopsy instruments: microhook scissors with single-action jaws (1); Blakesley dissecting and biopsy forceps (2); scissors with long, sharp, curved, double-action jaws (3); and scissors with serrated, curved, double-action jaws (4). (*C*) Probes: distendable palpation probe (1), palpation probe with cm markings (2), and irrigation and suction cannula (3). (*Courtesy of* Stephen J. Divers, Athens, GA.)

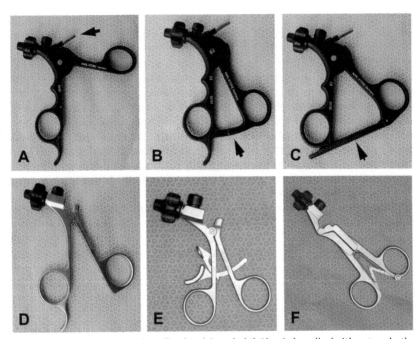

Fig. 16. Endoscopy instrument handles (Karl Storz). (*A*) Plastic handle (without racket) with radiosurgery connector (*arrow*). (*B*) Plastic handle with hemostat-style racket (*arrow*). (*C*) Plastic handle with Mahnes-style racket (*arrow*). (*D*) Metal handle without racket or radiosurgery connection. (*E*) Metal handle with disengageable racket but no radiosurgical connection. (*F*) Metal Y-handle with spring action. (*Courtesy of* Stephen J. Divers, Athens, GA.)

interchangeably with a variety of different handles (**Fig. 16**). Most handles are of plastic or metal construction and possess a radiosurgical connection that can turn scissors or forceps into monopolar devices. An optional hemostat or Mahnes-style racket mechanism is available to maintain firm hold of tissue even if the endoscopist releases their grip on the handle (see **Fig. 16**B, C, and E).

In human and domestic animal endosurgery, tilting tables are used to modify patient positioning and create advantageous organ displacement during surgery. The author modified the original design by the late Dr Ty Tankersley to develop a tilting table

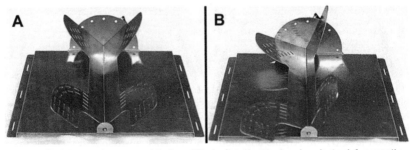

Fig. 17. Small tilting endoscopy table (modified after the Tankersley design) for reptiles and small mammals. (*Left*) Standard position to permit the animal to be restrained in dorsal recumbency. (*Right*) Table tilted by 30° to facilitate organ displacement and improved visualization of the dorsolateral structures. (*Courtesy of* Stephen J. Divers, Athens, GA.)

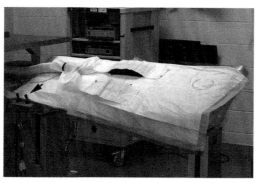

Fig. 18. Electronic tilting table with joystick control (*arrow*). (*Courtesy of* Stephen J. Divers, Athens, GA.)

capable of rotating small exotic patients from 30° to 90° from the midline (**Fig. 17**). In addition, joystick-controlled tilting surgery tables (**Fig. 18**) are helpful but expensive and likely to be limited to teaching hospitals and other referral institutions. Practitioners can probably achieve similar effects, albeit with more effort and less versatility, by using various positioning aids.

REFERENCES

1. Lhermette P, Sobel D. An introduction to endoscopy and endosurgery. In: Lhermette P, Sobel D, editors. BSAVA manual of canine and feline endoscopy and endosurgery. Cheltenham (England): British Small Animal Veterinary Association; 2008. p. 1–10.
2. AVMA. U.S. Pet Ownership & Demographics Sourcebook. American Veterinary Medical Association; 2007. Available at: http://www.avma.org/reference/marketstats/ownership.asp. Accessed December 12, 2009.
3. Tams TR. Small animal endoscopy. 2nd edition. St Louis (MO): Mosby; 1999. 497.
4. McCarthy TC. Veterinary endoscopy for the small animal practitioner. St Louis (MO): Elsevier; 2005. 624.
5. Taylor M. Endoscopic examination and biopsy techniques. In: Ritchie BW, Harrison GJ, Harrison LR, editors. Avian medicine: principles and application. Fort Worth (FL): Harrison Bird Diets International; 1994. p. 327–54.
6. Chamness CJ. Introduction to veterinary endoscopy and endoscopic instrumentation. In: McCarthy TC, editor. Veterinary endoscopy for the small animal practitioner. St louis (MO): Elsevier; 2004. p. 1–29.
7. Chamness CJ. Equipment for the avian and exotic endoscopist. Semin Avian Exotic Pet Med 1999;8:102–6.
8. Hernandez-Divers SJ. Endosurgical debridement and diode laser ablation of lung and air sac granulomas in psittacine birds. J Avian Med Surg 2002;16: 138–45.
9. Hernandez-Divers SJ. Diode laser surgery: principles and application in exotic animals. Semin Avian Exotic Pet Med 2002;11:208–20.
10. Hernandez-Divers SJ. Minimally-invasive endoscopic surgery of birds. J Avian Med Surg 2005;19(2):107–20.
11. Ternamian AM, Deitel M. Endoscopic threaded imaging port (EndoTIP) for laparoscopy: experience with different body weights. Obes Surg 1999;9:44–7.

Avian Diagnostic Endoscopy

Stephen J. Divers, BVetMed, DZooMed, DACZM, DipECZM(herp), FRCVS

KEYWORDS

• Avian • Minimally invasive • Endoscopy • Biopsy • Diagnosis

There are over 10,000 species of birds that vary tremendously in their anatomic, physiologic, and ecological adaptations. It would be impossible to cover all species; therefore this article has been purposefully restricted to those likely to be encountered in zoologic companion animal practice, namely the psittacines (parrots), passerines (song birds), raptors (birds of prey), and waterfowl (ducks and geese).

Avian endoscopy dates back several decades. The first published report of which the author is aware appeared in 1978 and described the evaluation of gonads in conscious birds.[1] Since that time, continued progress and refinement of human pediatric cystoscopy equipment resulted in the development of a dedicated avian endoscopy system.[2] Indeed, it is this avian system that was later used for reptiles, and fish. This telescope and operating sheath system facilitate examination and biopsy of internal organs via a single, small surgical incision. The benefits are minimally invasive internal examination, ability to safely perform biopsy procedures, and avoidance of invasive, lengthy surgery.

Avian veterinarians have been performing endoscopic assessments of the avian reproductive tract for many years, and despite the advent of DNA probes for sex identification of many species, clinicians involved with aviculturists, wholesalers, or retailers may still be asked to perform "surgical sexing". The ability to exploit the air sac system of birds enables the endoscopist to visualize most, if not all, of the major organs of clinical interest including liver, lung, air sac, heart, kidney, adrenal gland, spleen, pancreas, and reproductive and intestinal tracts. In addition, the oral approach permits examination of the buccal cavity, esophagus, crop (if present), proventriculus, ventriculus, glottis and trachea down to the level of the syrinx. The vent approach permits examination of the cloaca, and openings to the shell gland and ureters. This article has been written with the general practitioner in mind, and only the most commonly employed avian techniques have been described. For more detailed descriptions, the reader should consult the references.[2,3]

PATIENT SELECTION

Psittacines and passerines, as prey animals, generally mask signs of disease until advanced, while stoic raptors may continue to feed despite severe illness. In any

Department of Small Animal Medicine & Surgery (Zoological Medicine), College of Veterinary Medicine, University of Georgia, 501 DW Brooks Drive, Athens, GA 30602, USA
E-mail address: sdivers@uga.edu

Vet Clin Exot Anim 13 (2010) 187–202
doi:10.1016/j.cvex.2010.01.002

case, disease often is advanced by the time of presentation, and to further complicate matters, sick birds tend to deteriorate quickly. The most common endoscopic procedures performed by the author include coelioscopy (via the air sac system) with visceral biopsy, tracheoscopy, cloacoscopy, ingluvioscopy, and gastroscopy. Most of these procedures are single-entry diagnostic techniques, and they frequently conclude with the collection of samples for laboratory analyses. Most of the procedures described (or necessary modifications thereof) can be undertaken in most birds assuming equipment can be matched to patient size. The benefits of endoscopy are numerous but in most cases center on the fact that traditional approaches are far more invasive and carry significantly greater risks of morbidity and mortality (eg, syringeal tracheoscopy versus syringotomy, coelioscopy versus coeliotomy). In addition, the means to a definitive diagnosis relies upon the demonstration of a host pathologic response and the causative agent. Given the relative paucity of serologic tests available for most companion birds, combined with the 2- to 3-week delay in obtaining paired rising titers, the collection of tissue samples often represents the most expedient means, short of necropsy, for reaching a diagnosis. With the ability to examine internally and collect tissue samples, accurate ante-mortem diagnoses and hence treatment success have increased considerably. The concept of diagnosing and treating regional/organ disease (eg, respiratory disease, liver disease) based solely upon nonpathognomonic clinical signs, nonspecific imaging, hematology and biochemistry is largely outdated and difficult to justify given the current ease and widespread use of endoscopy in birds.

CONTRAINDICATIONS

Given the application of the 2.7 mm system, and more recent developments using 2 and 3 mm human pediatric equipment, the greatest limiting factor is probably the small size of most companion birds in combination with one's abilities as an endoscopist. In most cases, birds present with advanced disease, and therefore come with inherently higher risks that require critical management before anesthesia. In addition to poor medical status and anesthetic complications, small patient size often presents the greatest challenge. Obesity is often an issue in caged birds fed a high fat (seed) diet and can complicate both entry and evaluation, while reproductively active hens can present with large ovaries or eggs that reduce the working space within the coelom. Ascites is especially problematic, because lateral coelioscopy can create a connection between the hepatoperitoneal cavity and the air sac system, essentially drowning the bird.

INSTRUMENTATION

Given the variation in size and the nature of the procedures that may be performed, consideration should be given the correct selection of telescope and instruments (see the article by Stephen J. Divers elsewhere in this issue for further explanation of this topic). For most practices, the 2.7 mm system offers the greatest versatility, which can be built upon as individual practice caseload dictates. This system offers several advantages including simple single-entry access, ports for air or saline infusion, and an operating channel for the introduction of 1.7 mm instruments. In addition, the 1.9 mm telescope with integrated sheath (that can accommodate 1 mm instruments) and the 1 mm semirigid miniscope are useful for smaller birds. For multiple-entry endoscopy, the use of 2 and 3 mm human pediatric instruments has enabled coelomic endosurgery to become a reality in medium-to-large birds.[4,5]

PATIENT EVALUATION

Knowledge of avian anatomy and physiology, species-specific husbandry, and nutritional requirements are vital to properly evaluate the management and medical history of the patient. Inexperienced clinicians are directed to reviews on the subject and should prepare ahead of time.[6] Detailed anamnesis and complete physical examination, including accurate body weight, are essential, but may require sedation or anesthesia for untamed or stressed individuals. Serial clinicopathologic data can be helpful to quantify dehydration and may indicate infection and organ damage or dysfunction. Published reference ranges, however, are often broad and poorly sensitive or specific unless the bird is severely abnormal. In general, clinicopathologic and weight data collected at prior health examinations are most useful when assessing the individual bird. Complete blood counts and biochemistry panels are recommended, and even in birds weighing less than 30 g, hematocrit and total solids still can be obtained.

PATIENT PREPARATION

Most sick birds present dehydrated and anorectic. Fluid therapy, nutritional support, hospitalization in a warm incubator, and other nursing measures often are required to stabilize the patient before anesthesia and endoscopy. Rehydration using balanced crystalloid fluids (eg, Norm-R, lactated Ringer's solution) is recommended, and may be given intravenously or intraosseously for critical cases, or subcutaneously or orally for those more stable. Hypotensive birds should receive colloids (eg, hetastarch). Nutritional support varies, but for passerines and psittacines, crop tubing using a dedicated avian hand-rearing or critical care formula is effective. Raptors may eat whole, flayed, or chopped mice, rats, or chicks. Anorectic raptors can be crop-fed Hills a/d or other carnivore support diet in the immediate short term.

Fasting should be in accordance with body size and feeding strategy, and concentrate on emptying the crop (when present). For example, the smallest birds (eg, finches, budgerigars) should be fasted for no more than 30 to 60 minutes, and small-to-medium birds (eg, lovebirds, cockatiels) can be fasted for 1 to 2 hours. Medium-to-large birds (eg, African grays, Amazons, cockatoos, macaws) for 3 to 6 hours, while most raptors (eg, red-tailed hawk, great-horned owl) can be fasted for 6 to 12 hrs.

ANESTHESIA AND MONITORING

General anesthesia is recommended for all endoscopy procedures to avoid risking damage to equipment, patient, or staff. Previous suggestions that procedures can be performed in conscious birds are no longer acceptable.[1] Most birds are induced using isoflurane or sevoflurane by face mask, intubated using an uncuffed endotracheal tube, and maintained on gas. Positive pressure ventilation is valuable, and the author routinely connects all avian patients to a pressure cycle ventilator (Small Animal Ventilator, Vetronics, West Lafayette, IN, USA).[7] Respiratory rate, heart rate, end-tidal capnography, pulse oximetry, Doppler ultrasound, and temperature are monitored. Maintenance of temperature around 39° to 40°C (102° to 104°F) is important but difficult without using a combination of warm water and air blankets and appropriate plastic drapes. Vascular access and intraoperative fluid therapy at 10 mL/kg/h also is recommended using peripheral venous (ulnar, medial metatarsal) or intraosseous (distal ulnar, tibiotarsal) catheters.

Birds should be monitored closely on recovery, especially at the time of extubation. There remains controversy concerning the best use of opiates and other analgesics in birds, and taxa-specific effects have been documented; however, the author uses butorphanol (1 to 2 mg/kg) and meloxicam (0.5 mg/kg) routinely for all species.[8–10]

DIAGNOSTIC PROCEDURES

The general handling techniques used in avian endoscopy are similar to those employed for domesticated animals. The fact that most companion birds weigh less than 1 kg, however, requires careful control with the base of the telescope, eyepiece, and camera supported using the superior hand and the terminal end held by thumb and forefinger of the inferior hand.

Tracheoscopy

The lower respiratory tract can be evaluated using the left and right approaches to the air sacs and lungs. To complete the respiratory examination, however, an oral approach to the choana, trachea, and syrinx, and an external approach to the nares are required. Parrots that are severely dyspneic, or suddenly lose their voice and present in acute respiratory distress must first be stabilized. Oxygen, and when necessary, an air sac tube to provide an alternative airway, should be considered. Gas anesthesia can be delivered by an air sac tube leaving the mouth and trachea clear for endoscopy, biopsy, and debridement. In larger birds, the 3.5 mm protection sheath should be used and will enable tracheoscopy of birds over 400 to 500 g (eg, Amazons, African grays, macaws, and cockatoos). In smaller birds, a 1.0 mm semirigid endoscope or 1.9 mm telescope is required. The 1.9 mm and 2.7 mm telescopes can be used without any sheath; however, the advantages of reduced diameter should be weighed against increased risks of telescope damage. The bird is positioned in dorsal or ventral recumbency with the head and neck extended, and the telescope can be inserted through the glottis and advanced down the trachea (**Fig. 1**). A surgical plane of anesthesia is required to prevent coughing, but irritation and mucosal damage can be reduced by raising the leading edge of the 30° telescope above the mucosal surface while advancing down the trachea. The complete tracheal rings, syrinx, and sometimes even the proximal primary bronchi can be examined (**Fig. 2A–C**). Even where tracheal diameter prevents the use of a sheathed telescope, retrieval and biopsy forceps can be inserted alongside the telescope for retrieval of foreign bodies, debridement, and sample collection (**Fig. 2D–F**).

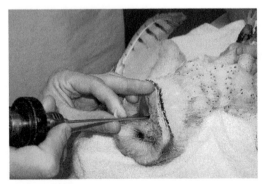

Fig. 1. Barn owl positioned in dorsal recumbency with head and neck extended for tracheoscopy using a 2.7 mm telescope without a sheath. (*Courtesy of* Stephen J. Divers, Athens, GA.)

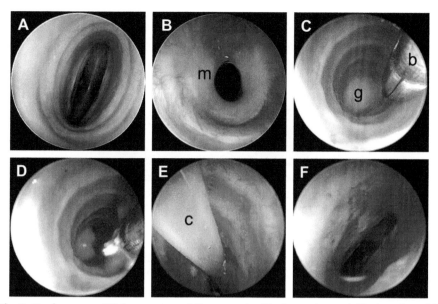

Fig. 2. Tracheoscopy. (*A*) Appearance of the normal psittacine syrinx and distal trachea. (*B*) Acquired tracheal membrane or stricture (m) in an African gray parrot presumably caused by prior traumatic intubation. (*C*) Syringeal granuloma (g) in a moluccan cockatoo. Biopsy forceps (b) are being advanced in preparation for sampling and debridement, while anesthesia is maintained via an airsac tube. (*C*) Endoscopic debridement of the same granuloma using 1.7 mm biopsy forceps inserted, not through the operating channel of a sheath, but rather alongside the telescope. (*D*) Following debridement, antimicrobial medication is delivered directly to the syrinx using a 1.7 mm catheter (c). (*E*) Appearance of the same syrinx 2 days after surgery revealing patency and the resolving nature of the infection. (*Courtesy of* Stephen J. Divers, Athens, GA.)

Ingluvioscopy and Gastroscopy

Examination of the oral cavity, esophagus, crop, proventriculus, and ventriculus are possible in most birds under 400 to 500 g using the 2.7 mm telescope and 4.8 mm operating sheath, via an oral approach. In larger birds, the ventriculus only can be reached using flexible endoscopes (**Fig. 3**), a longer telescope, or by the introduction of the standard 2.7 mm × 18 cm rigid telescope through a temporary ingluviotomy (**Fig. 4**). Gas insufflation can be used to dilate and examine the esophagus, crop, and proventriculus for foreign bodies. Warm (39° to 40°C, 102° to 104°F) sterile saline irrigation, however, provides better visualization, superior mucosal detail, and helps dilate the tract as the sheath–telescope is advanced (**Fig. 5**). All birds should be intubated and placed at a 30° to 45° incline to reduce the risks of aspiration. Foreign bodies can be removed using retrieval forceps or wire basket devices.

Cloacoscopy

Cloacoscopy using warm saline irrigation is very rewarding and preferred for evaluating cloacal papillomas, coprodeum, urodeum (including the openings to the ureters and, in females, the distal uterus), bursa of Fabricius, and proctodeum (**Figs. 6** and **7**). Excessive cloacal fluid administration can result in oral regurgitation, and so intubation remains important. Proliferative lesions can be biopsied easily, but care is required not

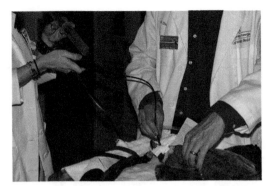

Fig. 3. Endoscopy of the upper gastrointestinal tract in large birds, like this hyacinth macaw, can be accomplished using flexible endoscopes or longer telescopes. (*Courtesy of* Stephen J. Divers, Athens, GA.)

to penetrate the cloacal wall.[11] Cloacal neoplasia can be ablated using radiosurgical or diode laser probes introduced via the instrument channel of the sheath (see **Fig. 7**).

Coelioscopy

There are four basic approaches to the coelom: left, right, ventral, and interclavicular. Physical examination, diagnostic imaging (including radiography and ultrasonography), and clinical pathology should be conducted to identify the most appropriate approach. For example, the spleen is best visualized via a left approach, the psittacine pancreas from the right, and both liver lobes only can be seen from a ventral approach. Most approaches to the avian coelom involve entry into and examination from within the air sacs. Therefore, it is important to keep sheath ports closed to avoid anesthetic compromise. In addition, left and right approaches should be avoided in birds with ascites, because fluid leakage into the air sac system is almost unavoidable; however, in such cases, a ventral midline approach between the airsacs is practical.

Left approach
The most commonly employed procedure involves a left approach into the air sac system, because male and female reproductive organs always can be seen (only

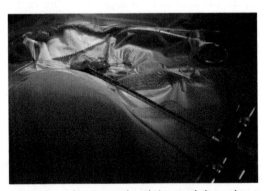

Fig. 4. The 2.7 mm telescope with 4.8 mm sheath inserted through a temporary ingluviotomy to examine the proventriculus and ventriculus of a macaw parrot. (*Courtesy of* Stephen J. Divers, Athens, GA.)

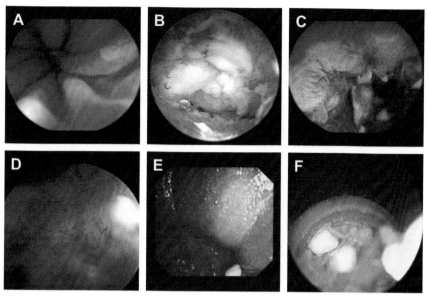

Fig. 5. Upper gastrointestinal endoscopy. (*A*) Appearance of the normal crop in an African gray parrot (2.7 mm telescope, saline infusion). (*B*) Severe crop candidiasis, indicated by the obvious white caseous debris, in a peregrine falcon (2.7 mm telescope, saline infusion). (*C*) Appearance of the normal proventriculus in an Amazon parrot. Note the obvious gastric glands and food debris within the lumen (2.7 mm telescope, saline infusion). (*D*) Ulcerated and inflamed proventriculus in a hyacinth macaw that presented with foreign carpet material within the ventriculus (2.7 mm telescope, saline infusion). (*E*) Appearance of the normal ventriculus in a scarlet macaw. Note the green koilin layer of the muscular ventriculus (3.8 mm flexible endoscope, air insufflation). (*F*) Rubber tube foreign body within the ventriculus of an African gray parrot that presented with chronic vomiting (2.7 mm telescope, saline infusion). (*Courtesy of* Stephen J. Divers, Athens, GA.)

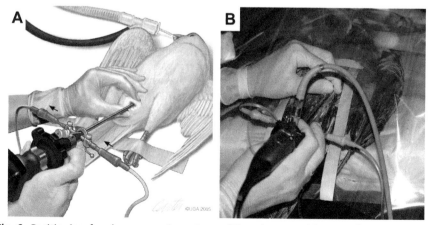

Fig. 6. Positioning for cloacoscopy in a pigeon (*A*) and macaw (*B*). Note the use of sterile saline infusion via the ports on the 4.8 mm operating sheath to control ingress and egress flow (*A, arrows*). (*Courtesy of* Stephen J. Divers, Athens, GA.)

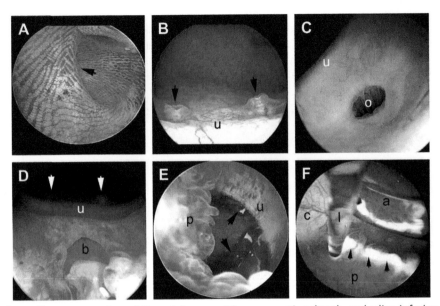

Fig. 7. Cloacoscopy using a 2.7 mm telescope, 4.8 mm operating sheath, and saline infusion. (*A*) Appearance of the normal coprodeum in a pigeon, with the opening to the rectum and large intestine shown (*arrow*). In psittacines, this opening is from the other side of the coprodeum. (*B*) Ureteral openings (*arrows*) and dorsal urodeal fold (u) in a pigeon. (*C*) Vaginal opening (o) close to the dorsolateral urodeal fold (u) in an immature red-tailed hawk. (*D*) Distal to the ureteral openings (*arrows*) and dorsal to the urodeal fold (u) lies the bursa of Fabricius (b), which is far more obvious in younger birds and involutes during maturation. (*E*) Papillomas (p) in a blue and gold macaw obscuring one side of the urodeal fold (u). Feces (*arrows*) can be seen entering the coprodeum. (*F*) Diode laser ablation of a large solitary papilloma (p) using a 600 μm fiber (l) in noncontact mode to coagulate the neoplastic tissue (*arrows*). Note the normal coprodeal mucosa (c) and the reflection from an air bubble (a). (*Courtesy of* Stephen J. Divers, Athens, GA.)

a few species have bilateral ovaries). The bird is positioned in right lateral recumbency with wings secured dorsad over the bird's back using self-adhesive tape. The left pelvic limb is pulled craniad and secured to the neck, again using self-adhesive bandage, to expose the left flank (**Fig. 8**A). The entry site is located immediately behind the last rib, and just ventral to the flexor cruris medialis muscle as it courses from caudal stifle to ischium (**Fig. 8**B). Very few feathers, if any, need to be plucked before aseptic preparation of the area. Following a 2 to 4 mm skin incision, straight hemostats, directed in a slight craniodorsal direction, are used to bluntly dissect between the thin subcutaneous tissues and enter the left caudal thoracic air sac. The hemostats are replaced by the sheathed telescope, and correct position within the caudal thoracic air sac is confirmed by the identification of lung (straight ahead), cranial thoracic air sac (left), abdominal air sac (right), caudal edge of liver and proventriculus (ventral), and ribs and intercostal muscles (dorsal) (**Fig. 9**).

Exploration of adjacent air sacs is accomplished by pressing the tip of the telescope against the air sac membrane and advancing the telescope in a sweeping motion until the air sac membranes are breached. Normal membranes are transparent and tissues in the adjacent air sac can be visualized and avoided. Great care is required when breaking through thickened, opaque air sacs, because vision is impaired and visceral

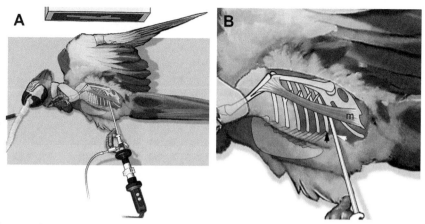

Fig. 8. (*A*) Positioning a macaw for left lateral coelioscopy. The left pelvic limb is pulled craniad and taped to the neck macaw to expose the left flank. (*B*) Telescope (*white arrow*) entry is just behind the last rib (*black arrow*), at the ventral border of the flexor cruris medialis muscle (m). (*Courtesy of* Stephen J. Divers, Athens, GA.)

trauma can occur if the telescope is blindly advanced. Lung, liver, heart, and associated great vessels can be examined from the cranial thoracic air sac (see **Fig. 9**), while urogenital, intestinal, splenic, adrenal gland, and associated vasculature can be visualized from the abdominal air sac (**Figs. 10–13**).

There is no need to repair the small holes punctured in the air sac membranes, as they generally heal within 5 to 10 days. Postoperative subcutaneous emphysema may be seen in some birds when only skin closure is performed. Therefore, either a single absorbable (eg, poliglecaprone 25) suture that incorporates both muscle and skin, or a two-layer closure is recommended.

Right approach

The right approach is essentially the same as previously described. Of particular note is the asymmetrical location of the psittacine pancreas, which can be accessed most easily from the right abdominal air sac in most species by following the duodenum (most caudal intestinal loop) caudoventrad (see **Fig. 13**).

Ventral approach

The ventral approach provides excellent access to both left and right liver lobes. In cases of ascites, the ventral approach is preferred, because the telescope can enter the hepatoperitoneal cavity without entering the air sac system. The bird is positioned in dorsal recumbency, and following aseptic preparation, entry is made in the ventral midline, just caudal to the keel (**Fig. 14**). The hepatoperitoneal cavity is divided into left and right sides, and the midline membrane can be perforated as previously described.

Clavicular approach

In order to identify and preserve the crop, a larger surgical approach (1 cm) is required in the midventral coelomic inlet. Upon entering the clavicular air sac, the telescope must be advanced carefully because of the close proximity of left and right brachiocephalic branches and other major vessels in this region. The clavicular approach is used less commonly but does provide access to the syringeal region, heart, and great vessels, and has been useful for the identification, sampling, and treatment of cranial coelomic masses (**Fig. 15**).[12]

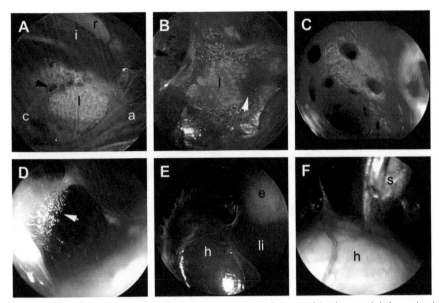

Fig. 9. Coelioscopy using a 2 .7 mm telescope. (*A*) View from within the caudal thoracic air-sac in a pigeon. The ventrolateral aspect of the lung (l) and the primary ostium (*arrow*) lie directly ahead, with the ribs (r) and intercostal muscles (i) above. The cranial thoracic (c) and abdominal (a) airsacs lie to the left and right, respectively. (*B*) View from within the caudal thoracic airsac of an amazon parrot with hemorrhage (*white arrow*) within the left lung (l). The opening to the primary ostium (*black arrow*) is also visible. (*C*) View within the primary ostium of the caudal thoracic air sac demonstrating the normal appearance of parabronchi and lung tissue in a pigeon. (*D*) View of the primary ostium of the cranial thoracic air sac of a macaw with severe dyspnea. Note the fungal mycelia (*arrow*), which on biopsy, proved to be *Aspergillus fumigatus*. (*E*) Normal appearance of the heart (h), liver (li), and distal esophagus (e) from within the cranial thoracic air sac of an Amazon parrot. (*F*) View of the heart with grossly thickened and opaque pericardium (h) in an Amazon parrot that presented with peripheral weakness and lethargy. Endoscopic scissors (s) were used to create a large pericardial window to aid cardiac function, and pericardial biopsy confirmed the diagnosis as constrictive fibrosing pericarditis. (*Courtesy of* Stephen J. Divers, Athens, GA.)

Biopsy Technique

One of the greatest benefits of endoscopy is that when an abnormal structure or pathologic lesion is observed, biopsies can be taken under direct visual control. Biopsies can be harvested from the kidneys, gonads, liver, spleen, pancreas, lung, fat, air sac, coelomic musculature, and, in general, any abnormal soft tissue structure. It is important to examine as much of the target structure as possible to determine whether pathology is focal, multifocal or diffuse. In cases of diffuse renal or hepatic disease (eg, tubulonephrosis, nephrocalcinosis, hepatic lipidosis, hepatitis), two or three biopsies taken from the most convenient sites are generally diagnostic. Ultrasound-guided and blind-percutaneous biopsy techniques may be equally effective in diagnosing diffuse disease. However, poorer visualization of closely associated structures makes iatrogenic trauma more likely. Most diagnostic failures occur because of poor tissue selection for biopsy, and this is especially true when dealing with focal (eg, abscess, neoplasm, cyst) and multifocal diseases (eg, pyogranulomata, mycobacteriosis). In these cases, direct endoscopic visualization offers the best chance of sampling the

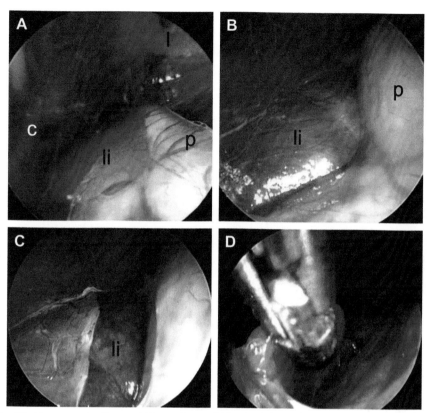

Fig. 10. Liver examination and biopsy from within the left caudal thoracic air sac. (*A*) View of the normal liver (li), proventriculus (p), lung (l), and cranial thoracic air sac (c) in a pigeon. (*B*) View of the swollen and discolored liver (li), and distended proventriculus in a black palm cockatoo with chlamydophilosis. (*C*) In preparation for biopsy, the ventral floor of the caudal thoracic air sac and the hepatoperitoneal membranes have been incised using 1.3 mm scissors to expose the liver parenchyma (li). (*D*) 1.7 mm biopsy forceps are advanced through this incision to collect a liver sample. (*Courtesy of* Stephen J. Divers, Athens, GA.)

most appropriate area(s). In cases of focal or multifocal disease, single or multiple discrete lesions are visible, and biopsies ideally should be harvested from the edge of the lesion taking normal and abnormal tissue in the same biopsy sample for both microbiology and histology. Alternatively, and technically easier, small biopsies can be collected from the abnormal and normal areas and submitted together for comparison. Focal disease deep within an organ showing no surface lesions, although rare, may be missed on endoscopic examination. It is important to correlate biopsy histopathology and microbiology with clinicopathologic data when dealing with organ disease. It is often surprising how biopsy results provide a definitive diagnosis even in the face of unremarkable clinicopathologic data.

When confronted by a potentially cystic lesion or abscess, it is safer to first attempt drainage using fine needle aspiration, rather than risk leakage into the air sacs or coelom. When attempting to take a liver or lung biopsy, it is preferable to first incise the air sac and serosal membranes using endoscopic scissors. This provides better access to the tissue parenchyma and yields biopsies of superior histologic quality

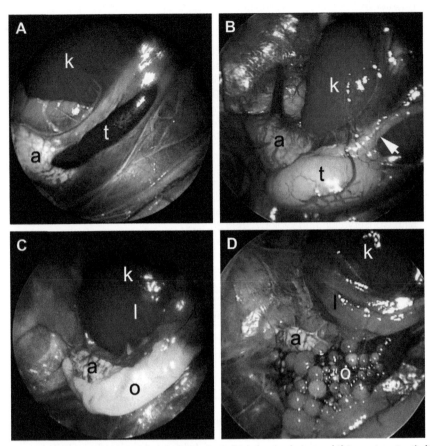

Fig. 11. Gonadal examination from within the left abdominal air sac. (*A*) Immature testis (t), adrenal gland (a), and cranial division of the kidney (k) in a moluccan cockatoo. (*B*) Mature testis (t), vas deferens (*arrow*), adrenal gland (a), and cranial division of the kidney (k) in an Amazon parrot. (*C*) Immature ovary (o), suspensory ligament (l), adrenal gland (a), and cranial division of the kidney (k) in an African gray parrot. (*D*) Mature, quiescent ovary (o), suspensory ligament (l), adrenal gland, and cranial division of the kidney (k) in an umbrella cockatoo. (*Courtesy of* Stephen J. Divers, Athens, GA.)

with minimal artifacts. Biopsies of the spleen, kidney, testis, adrenal gland and most pathologic lesions usually can be taken without the use of scissors. Postsampling hemorrhage tends to be minor and inconsequential thanks to the avian extrinsic coagulation pathway, and in particular, tissue-associated thromboplastin.[11–13]

Liver biopsy

In cases of diffuse liver pathology, the most accessible sampling site from a lateral approach is the caudal edge of the liver, located on the ventral floor of the caudal thoracic air sac. To access the liver, it is necessary to incise the air sac and hepatoperitoneal membranes using scissors. The scissors are opened, and the fixed blade is inserted gently through the membranes parallel with the caudal edge of the liver. While keeping the blades open, the scissors-sheath-telescope unit is elevated and

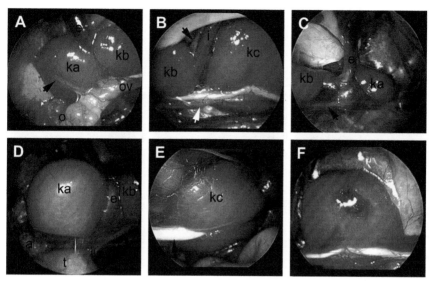

Fig. 12. Renal examination and biopsy from within the abdominal air sac. (*A*) External iliac vein (e) running between the cranial (ka) and middle (kb) divisions of the left kidney. Note the close association of the ovary (o), suspensory ligament (arrow), and oviduct (ov). (*B*) Ischiatic vein (i) and spinal nerves (*black arrow*) running between the middle (kb) and caudal (kc) divisions of the left kidney, with the ureter and immature oviduct (*white arrow*) ventromediad. (*C*) Abnormally small cranial (ka) and middle (kb) divisions of the right kidney in a macaw. The external iliac vein (e) and ureter (*arrow*) are also shown. Such anomalies can be congenital or the result of chronic disease and renal fibrosis. (*D*) Swollen cranial division of the left kidney (ka) in an Amazon parrot causing caudal displacement of the external iliac vein (e). Biopsy confirmed bacterial glomerulonephritis. The middle division of the kidney (kb), adrenal gland (a), and testis (t) are also visible. (*E*) Renomegaly of the caudal divisions of both kidneys (kc) and dilation of the ureters (*arrow*) associated with lead intoxication and renal tubular necrosis in a macaw. (*F*) Caudal division of the kidney following biopsy using 1.7 mm biopsy forceps. Note the minor hemorrhage that typically stops quickly thanks to tissue-bound thromboplastin. (*Courtesy of* Stephen J. Divers, Athens, GA.)

advanced to extend the incision. Once the incision is large enough to permit the introduction of biopsy forceps, the blades are closed and the scissors retracted. Biopsy forceps then are inserted through the incision, and a clean liver sample can be collected (see **Fig. 10**). Multiple biopsies can be taken from the same site. Biopsy without first incising the membranes overlying the liver tends to result in greater biopsy artifact.

Kidney biopsy

Renal biopsies can be collected from the cranial, middle, or caudal divisions of the kidney from within the abdominal air sacs. In general, there is no need to use scissors, as the renal parenchyma protrudes and is accessed easily with minimal artifact (see **Fig. 12**).

Lung biopsy

Lung tissue is most accessible from within the left or right caudal thoracic air sacs. The air sac and pleural membranes first must be incised using scissors. It is generally

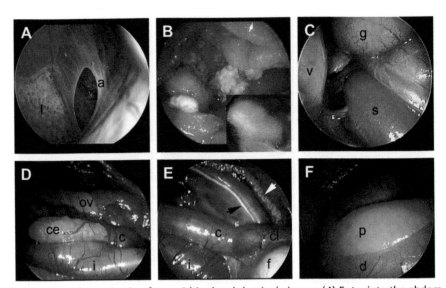

Fig. 13. Visceral examination from within the abdominal air sacs. (*A*) Entry into the abdominal air sac is achieved by gently forcing the telescope through the interface between the caudal thoracic and abdominal airsacs (a). Lung (l) is also visible. (*B*) View of grossly thickened air sacs and fungal mycelia (insert) associated with aspergillosis in an Amazon parrot. (*C*) View of the pigeon spleen (s) and the closely associated gonad (g) and ventriculus (v). (*D*) View of the oviduct (ov), small intestinal tract (i), colon (c), and one of two small ceca (ce) from within the left abdominal airsac of a pigeon. (*E*) View of the cloaca (cl), colon (c), cloacal fat pad (f), ureter (*black arrow*), vas deferens (*white arrow*), and small intestine (i) of an Amazon parrot. (*F*) View of the pancreas (p) and duodenal loop (d) from within the right abdominal air sac of a macaw. (*Courtesy of* Stephen J. Divers, Athens, GA.)

easier to rotate the scissors within the operating channel, such that the fixed blade is dorsal. The scissors-sheath-telescope unit is advanced, and the point of the fixed blade is inserted through the membranes covering the lung. The scissors-sheath-telescope unit is then gently moved ventrad, creating a dorsoventral incision through which biopsy forceps can be inserted to collect lung biopsies.

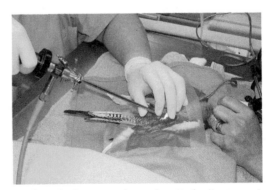

Fig. 14. Ventral approach to the hepatoperitoneal cavity for liver examination and biopsy in a cockatiel with ascites. (*Courtesy of* Stephen J. Divers, Athens, GA.)

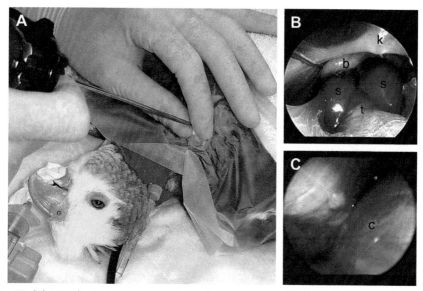

Fig. 15. (*A*) Interclavicular endoscopy in an Amazon parrot. (*B*) Normal appearance of the syringeal muscles (s), trachea (t), cranial keel (k), and brachiocephalic trunk (b) as seen from within the clavicular airsac of a pigeon. (*C*) Large cyst (c) associated with an adenocarcinoma of the cranial coelom as seen from within the clavicular airsac of an Amazon parrot. (*Courtesy of* Stephen J. Divers, Athens, GA.)

Splenic biopsy

The spleen is visualized best from within the left abdominal air sac, and although greater hemorrhage usually is associated with biopsy, the clinical consequences appear minimal.[11]

Pancreatic biopsy

Pancreatic biopsies are collected most easily from within the right abdominal air sac of psittacines.

COMPLICATIONS

The major complications encountered typically are associated with anesthesia and the advanced disease state of many birds at the time of presentation. The importance of stabilization and a thorough preoperative evaluation cannot be overemphasized. Endotracheal intubation, ventilation, intravenous or intraosseous catheterization with perioperative fluid support, and warm air/water blankets are important. Minor hemorrhage following tissue biopsy is common but insignificant. Most endoscopy issues are related to operator error until experience and ability have been gained. In general, the ability to examine birds internally and collect tissue samples greatly aids diagnosis and improves treatment success.

POSTOPERATIVE CARE

Birds should be supervised closely on recovery, as anesthetic compromise can ensue following extubation and cessation of cardiorespiratory support. Fluid therapy and nutritional support should continue, with psittacines and passerines eating within an hour of recovery. Meloxicam is used routinely postoperatively, although opiates and local anesthetics could prove useful as part of a balanced approach to analgesia. Typically birds return to normal function quickly following single-entry diagnostic procedures compared with more traditional, invasive surgery. Sutures are removed at 7 to 10 days if still present.

OUTCOME

Return to normal behaviors and weight gain is often the most useful indicator for improvement. Serial clinicopathology and imaging also can be useful if abnormalities were detected preoperatively. Serial endoscopic evaluations can be used to monitor patients, especially as some diseases (eg, hepatic lipidosis, glomerulonephrosis) may have a protracted course.

REFERENCES

1. Harrison GJ. Endoscopic examination of avian gonadal tissues. Vet Med Small Anim Clin 1978;73(4):479–84.
2. Taylor M. Endoscopic examination and biopsy techniques. In: Ritchie BW, Harrison GJ, Harrison LR, editors. Avian medicine: principles and application. Fort Worth (FL): Harrison Bird Diets International; 1994. p. 327–54.
3. Hernandez-Divers SJ, Hernandez-Divers SM. Avian diagnostic endoscopy. Comp Cont Educ Pract Vet 2004;26(11):839–52.
4. Hernandez-Divers SJ. Minimally-invasive endoscopic surgery of birds. J Avian Med Surg 2005;19(2):107–20.
5. Hernandez-Divers SJ, Stahl SJ, Wilson GH, et al. Endoscopic orchidectomy and salpingohysterectomy of pigeons (Columba livia): an avian model for minimally invasive endosurgery. J Avian Med Surg 2007;21(1):22–37.
6. Ritchie BW, Harrison GJ, Harrison LR. Avian medicine: principles and application. Fort Worth (FL): Harrison Bird Diets International; 1994. 327–54.
7. Touzot-Jourde G, Hernandez-Divers SJ, Trim CM. Cardiopulmonary effects of controlled versus spontaneous ventilation in pigeons anesthetized for coelioscopy. J Am Vet Med Assoc 2004;227(9):1424–8.
8. Sladky KK, Krugner-Higby L, Meek-Walker E, et al. Serum concentrations and analgesic effects of liposome-encapsulated and standard butorphanol tartrate in parrots. Am J Vet Res 2006;67(5):775–81.
9. Paul-Murphy J, Hess JC, Fialkowski JP. Pharmacokinetic properties of a single intramuscular dose of buprenorphine in African grey parrots (Psittacus erithacus erithacus). J Avian Med Surg 2004;18(4):224–8.
10. Paul-Murphy J, Ludders JW. Avian analgesia. Veterinary Clin North Am Exot Anim Pract 2001;4:35–45.
11. Hernandez-Divers SJ, Wilson GH, Lester VK, et al. Evaluation of coelioscopic splenic biopsy and cloacoscopic bursa of Fabricius biopsy techniques in pigeons (Columba livia). J Avian Med Surg 2006;20(4):234–41.
12. Hanley CS, Wilson GH, Latimer KS, et al. Interclavicular hemangiosarcoma in a double yellow headed Amazon (Amazona ochrocephala oratrix). J Avian Med Surg 2005;19(2):130–7.
13. Sturkie PD, Griminger P, Wilson GH, Latimer KS. Blood: physical characteristics, formed elements, hemoglobin and coagulation. In: Sturkie PD, editor. Avian physiology. New York: Springer-Verlag; 1976. p. 53–75.

Avian Endosurgery

Stephen J. Divers, BVetMed, DZooMed, DACZM, DipECZM(herp), FRCVS

KEYWORDS

• Avian • Minimally invasive • Surgery • Endoscopy

In the field of zoologic medicine, the application of diagnostic endoscopy has shown great promise in various species but probably has been exploited most by avian veterinarians.[1–3] Avian veterinarians routinely use endoscopy to evaluate the respiratory tract, gastrointestinal tract, and coelomic viscera, particularly the urogenital tract, liver, and kidneys.[4–7] Rigid endoscopy is used most commonly for diagnostic purposes in birds.[3,8] Most endoscopic systems use a rigid telescope housed within a sheath through which basic instruments can be inserted into the field of view. This technique has been extremely effective for visualization and biopsy but is severely limited in its ability to facilitate surgery where the triangulation of multiple instruments generally is required.

Avian endosurgery may be single-, double- or tripe-entry in nature. Single-entry techniques are similar to those employed for diagnostic evaluations and biopsy. They rely on the use of a single instrument inserted through the operating channel of the sheathed telescope, while double- and triple-entry techniques use two or three separate devices simultaneously. The practical application of single-entry diagnostic endoscopy is relatively straightforward. With appropriate training, veterinarians can quickly become proficient and use endoscopy to visualize internal organs and collect samples. This is thanks to the single-entry nature of the procedures, such that the instrument is used along a single plane (advance or retract) within the endoscopy field without the need to triangulate instruments independently from the telescope. Although this system has proven extremely effective for diagnosis, it has obvious drawbacks when attempting to perform endosurgical procedures, because forceps, scissors, retractors, and radiosurgery devices must be used independently within the endoscopy field. Trying to perform endosurgery through a single port is like trying to perform traditional surgery with one hand tied behind one's back. One needs two hands to use two independent instruments! So while the need for two or three independent ports is obvious, as soon as the instruments become independent of the telescope, it becomes necessary to triangulate (coordinate) instruments with the telescope. Consequently, the instrument is no longer restricted to the single plane within the operating sheath, but can be

Department of Small Animal Medicine & Surgery (Zoological Medicine), College of Veterinary Medicine, University of Georgia, 501 DW Brooks Drive, Athens, GA 30602, USA
E-mail address: sdivers@uga.edu

Vet Clin Exot Anim 13 (2010) 203–216
doi:10.1016/j.cvex.2010.01.003
1094-9194/10/$ – see front matter © 2010 Elsevier Inc. All rights reserved.

wielded in all three planes independent of the telescope, creating a second variable. If a second instrument is added, then there are three variables. There can be little doubt that using one or two instruments separate from the telescope raises the difficulty of endosurgery by at least an order of magnitude. Veterinarians who make the transition from single-entry diagnostic techniques to multiple-entry endosurgery tend to have most difficulty with

1. Multiple port placement—accurate anatomic knowledge and surgical placement of cannulae are essential (**Fig. 1**)
2. Instrument triangulation and depth perception—bringing two independent instruments into the endoscopy field of view and keeping them there and coordinated with the telescope takes practice (**Figs. 2** and **3**)
3. Reduced tactile feedback—tissue handling occurs at a greater distance, and it takes practice to appreciate how much force and tension can be applied (see **Fig. 3**)
4. Maintaining hemostasis—fortunately, radiosurgery units can be attached to various endoscopy instruments to assist with dissection and hemostasis.

Consequently, endosurgery can never be the ultrafast 2 minute procedure that many have become accustomed to when performing surgical sexing of birds. On the contrary, it demands far greater planning, preparation, patience, and perseverance. Once mastered, however, endosurgery opens up many opportunities to perform procedures with minimal trauma, with advantages well documented in human medicine.

PATIENT SELECTION

In addition to the general indications and contraindications for performing endoscopy in birds, there are some additional patient issues to consider before attempting

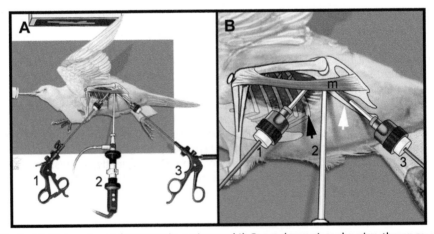

Fig. 1. Multiple-entry endosurgery in a pigeon. (*A*) General overview showing the approximate position of the forceps (1) for the left hand, telescope-camera (2) positioned in the middle and resting on a support aid, and monopolar radiosurgical scissors (3) for the right hand. (*B*) Close-up of the surgical area illustrating the anatomic position of the forceps (1), telescope (2), and scissors (3) in relation to the last rib (*black arrow*), pubis bone (*white arrow*), and flexor cruris medialis muscle (m). (*Courtesy of* Stephen J. Divers, Athens, GA.)

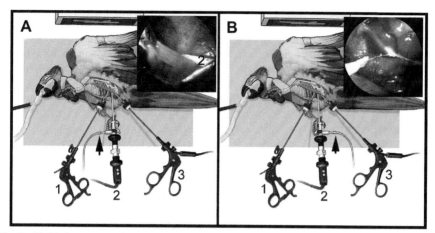

Fig. 2. Multiple-entry endosurgery in a macaw. The 30° oblique angle of the 2.7 mm telescope is particularly useful, because it enables the view within the coelom to be changed by simply rotating the telescope around its longitudinal axis. (*A*) With the light guide cable positioned to the left (*arrow*), the oblique view is directed caudad, and the distal uterus can be seen (insert). (*B*) With the light guide cable positioned to the right (*arrow*), the oblique view is directed craniad and the ovary can be seen. (*Courtesy of* Stephen J. Divers, Athens, GA.)

endosurgery. First and foremost, the issue of physical size remains. It is simply not going to be possible to fit a telescope and two independent instruments inside a budgerigar or cockatiel! The size of the patient remains a major limiting factor, and in small birds, single- or double-entry techniques may be all that are possible.

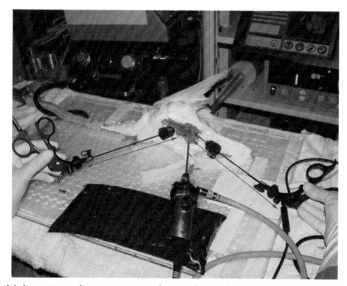

Fig. 3. Multiple-entry endosurgery to perform salpingohysterectomy in a research pigeon (the drape has been omitted for photography). Tactile feedback is diminished, because the surgeon is now more distant from the tissues that are being manipulated. (*Courtesy of* Stephen J. Divers, Athens, GA.)

CONTRAINDICATIONS

Given the availability of small telescopes (1.9 and 2.7 mm) and more recent developments in 2 to 3 mm human pediatric instrumentation, the greatest limiting factor is probably the small size of most companion birds in combination with the limited but evolving abilities of avian endosurgeons. In addition to anesthetic contraindications, gross obesity and ascites are common problems that strongly argue against endosurgery.

INSTRUMENTATION

Given the variation in size and the nature of the procedures that may be performed, consideration should be given to the correct selection of telescope and instruments. The basic rigid telescope system for avian veterinarians has been developed from human cystoscopy equipment.[9,10] Probably the most commonly used endoscope is the 30° Hopkins telescope, 2.7 mm × 18 cm, connected to a halogen or xenon light source via a fiber-optic cable (Karl Storz Veterinary Endoscopy America Inc, Goleta, CA, USA). The smaller 1.9 mm × 18 cm telescope and integrated sheath system is also available and is preferable for birds weighing less than 200 g. Endoscopy cameras and monitor display of the endoscopic field are essential for performing endosurgery.[8,11] The miniature endoscopy system originally designed for human pediatric laparoscopy is now marketed specifically for cats, small dogs and small exotic species (Karl Storz Veterinary Endoscopy America Inc), see the article by Stephen J. Divers elsewhere in this issue for further explanation of this topic.

Coelioscopy and endosurgery must be performed under general anesthesia using appropriate aseptic techniques and sterilized instruments. Equipment sterilization using hydrogen peroxide vapor or ethylene oxide gas is preferred, but cold sterilization using glutaraldehyde is acceptable. Operating room design and layout are important. An endovideo camera coupled to a monitor facing the surgeon at eye-level will greatly improve the endoscopist's ergonomics and surgical ability. Standard and endoscopic surgical equipment and supplies also should be arranged to be within easy reach.

PATIENT EVALUATION

Endosurgical procedures are more involved. Indeed total anesthesia and surgery times are likely to be greater than for a traditional surgical approach until the surgeon becomes competent with the endoscopic techniques. When first embarking upon endosurgery, it is wise to advise the client that the endoscopic procedure will be converted to a traditional surgical approach if necessary. In this way, the veterinarian can build an endoscopy caseload while retaining the right to convert if difficulties arise. Initially, surgeons often find themselves having to convert to a traditional approach early on in the procedure, but with each subsequent experience, they will advance further and further, until eventually the procedure is completed endoscopically.

PATIENT PREPARATION

The most common multiple-entry endosurgery performed by the author is salpingo-hysterectomy. Typically, birds initially present with some form of reproductive disease that following successful management are often pretreated with leuprolide acetate (700 to 800 µg/kg intramuscularly every 14 days for three treatments) before surgery.[12] This has the advantage of reducing the size and vascularity of the reproductive tract before endosurgery.

Unless anatomic or disease considerations dictate otherwise, a left approach to the avian coelom is preferred. For unfamiliar species, survey radiographs can be extremely helpful in determining the precise insertion points for additional ports. Some veterinarians prefer to extend the pelvic limb caudad and enter the coelom in front of the leg. Although this technique is suitable for single-entry endoscopy, it does not lend itself to multiple-entry procedures because of the restricted surgical field exposed. Positioning the limb craniad maximizes caudal flank exposure and facilitates additional port placement for double- and triple-entry techniques.

ANESTHESIA AND MONITORING

Given the degree of preparation required for telescope and cannula(e) placement, and that inexperience may initially result in longer surgery times, high-quality anesthesia and monitoring are essential. Preoperative stabilization and support are vital, and birds routinely should be intubated and ventilated. Body temperature must be monitored and maintained above 100°F using radiant heat sources, water-circulating blankets, or forced warm air heaters. Intravenous or intraosseous catheterization and intraoperative fluid support are the norm, and in larger birds, intra-arterial catheterization and direct blood pressure monitoring are preferred. Monitoring should be performed and recorded by a dedicated individual, and should include reflexes, muscle tone, eye position and corneal/palpebral reflexes, pulse oximetry, electrocardiogram (ECG), and end-tidal capnography.

SURGICAL PROCEDURES
Single-entry Techniques

Single-entry endosurgery is limited to a single instrument that cannot be manipulated independently of the telescope (**Fig. 4**). This technique provides surgical access to the heart, liver, spleen, gastro-intestinal and urogenital tracts via the cranial thoracic,

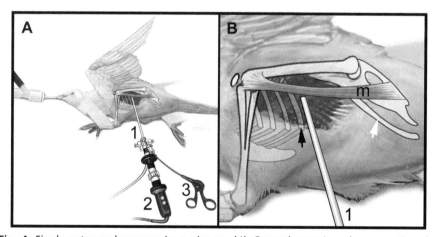

Fig. 4. Single-entry endosurgery in a pigeon. (*A*) General overview demonstrating the approximate position of the telescope (1), camera (2), and flexible instrument (3) inserted down the instrument channel of the operating sheath. (*B*) Close-up view of the surgical site illustrating the position of the telescope (1) to enter the caudal thoracic air sac, just caudal to the last rib (*black arrow*) and ventral to the flexor cruris medialis muscle (m). The pubis bone (*white arrow*) is also palpable and useful for orientation. (*Courtesy of* Stephen J. Divers, Athens, GA.)

caudal thoracic, or abdominal air sacs (see the article by Stephen J. Divers elsewhere in this issue for further explanation of this topic). Salpingohysterectomy has been described in juvenile cockatiels by using the 2.7 mm telescope, 4.8 mm operating sheath, and 1.7 mm grasping forceps to break down the suspensory ligaments and remove the infundibulum, oviduct, and uterus.[13] Completing this surgery required exteriorizing the reproductive tract through the single surgical entry site, with final crushing and transection of the uterus performed externally by a second surgeon. Additional hemostasis was not used, and despite some minor bleeding from the cloaca, there was no mortality or apparent morbidity associated with the procedure. This technique is better described as endoscope-assisted rather than truely endoscopic, because surgery was completed outside the coelom using standard surgical instruments. Nevertheless, endoscopy prevented the need for a more invasive coeliotomy and reduced surgical trauma. A greater risk of severe hemorrhage would be expected if this technique were used in mature hens because of the greater vascular supply and lack of effective endoscopic hemostasis.

Air sac granulomatas have been removed successfully in several parrots using a combination of endoscopic debridement and diode laser ablation.[11] Because of the avascular nature of the granulomata, debridement with 1.7 mm biopsy forceps was possible without additional hemostasis (**Fig. 5**). Diode laser was used to ablate and sterilize the infected areas. With this technique, resection is restricted to relatively small avascular masses. Hemostasis is more of a concern when dealing with larger, more vascular structures, while the small size of the biopsy forceps would result in excessively long debridement times.

Disadvantages of single-entry techniques include reliance on a single instrument, small size of a limited number of available instruments, and codependence between instrument and telescope. For small birds, however, single-entry techniques may provide the only practical alternative to standard coeliotomy.

Multiple-entry Procedures

Recently, the use of miniature endoscopic equipment, pioneered in human pediatric laparoscopy, has been applied to avian surgery.[14] The addition of a second and third operating port using 2.5 or 3.5 mm cannulae has facilitated the use of 2 or 3 mm instruments within the avian coelom. Triangulation of various instruments coupled with radiosurgical hemostasis has made several endoscopic procedures possible, including salpingohysterectomy, orchidectomy, and mass resection.[14,15] Endosurgical salpingohysterectomy and orchidectomy were developed using a pigeon model, and have subsequently been applied to psittacines and waterfowl in clinical practice.

Orchidectomy (double-entry technique)

Initial positioning and preparation are similar to those previously described for the left approach for coelioscopy (see the article by Stephen J. Divers elsewhere in this issue for further explanation of this topic). More feathers, however, are plucked from the left flank to reveal a surgical field that extends from the last intercostal space (cranial) to the pericloacal region (caudal), and from the dorsal border of the flexor cruris medialis muscle (dorsal) to the ventral border of the pubis bone (ventral). Following aseptic preparation, a 2 mm skin incision is made behind the last rib, or midway between the last rib and the pubis bone, at the ventral border of the flexor cruris medialis muscle. Blunt entry into the left abdominal air sac is achieved using straight hemostats. The 2.7 mm telescope housed within a 3.5 mm protection sheath is inserted into the left abdominal air sac. Following a brief examination to confirm the gender of the bird, the presence of a normal urogenital system, and a lack of any visible

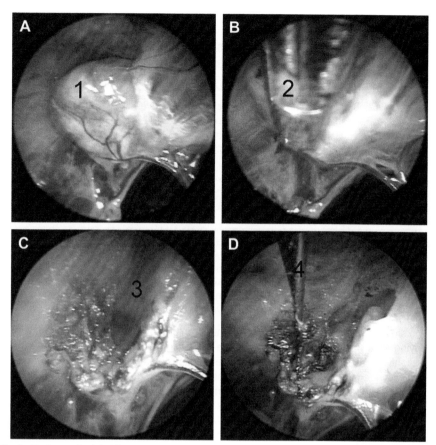

Fig. 5. Endoscopic debridement and diode laser ablation of a fungal granuloma (*Aspergillus fumigatus*) in the caudal thoracic air sac of a parrot. (*A*) Coelioscopic view of a fungal granuloma (1) attached to the lung and the caudodorsal aspect of the caudal thoracic air sac. (*B*) Debridement of the granuloma using 1.7 mm biopsy forceps (2). (*C*) Diode laser ablation of the remaining granuloma using a 600 μm fiber with precarbonized tip (3) at 3 W continuous power. (*D*) Local application of amphotericin B delivered using a fine aspiration/injection needle (4). (*Courtesy of* Stephen J. Divers, Athens, GA.)

pathology, a second port is created just behind the pubis bone, at the ventral border of the flexor cruris medialis muscle. This equates to approximately midway along the palpable pubis bone. A 3.5 mm cannula and trocar are inserted through a 2 mm skin incision, and, using gentle sustained axial pressure, are advanced into the caudal aspect of the left abdominal air sac under endoscopic guidance. Once inside the abdominal air sac, the trocar is removed and the cannula advanced 2 to 4 mm into the lumen of the air sac. The polypectomy snare attached to a radiofrequency unit (4.0 MHz Surgitron; Ellman International, Oceanside, NY, USA), set to an initial suggested power setting of 25% on cut and coagulation mode, is then inserted through the cannula and into the endoscopic field (**Fig. 6**). The telescope is rotated to provide a view of the testis, as seen from within the left abdominal air sac. The polypectomy snare is advanced, extended, and placed over the testis, taking care not to entrap any part of the cranial division of the kidney, adrenal gland, or vena cava.

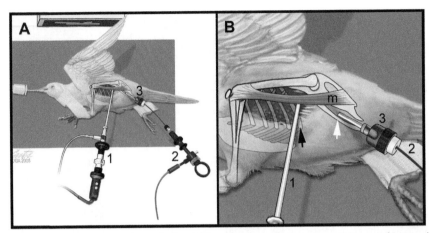

Fig. 6. (*A*) Double-entry endosurgical orchidectomy in a pigeon using a 2.7 mm telescope (1) and radiosurgical polypectomy snare (2) inserted through a 3.5 mm cannula (3). (*B*) Close-up view of the surgical site illustrating the entry of the 2.7 mm telescope (1) behind the last rib (*black arrow*) at the ventral border of the flexor curis medialis muscle (m). Insertion of the polypectomy snare (2) through a 3.5 mm cannula (3) positioned just caudal to midpubis bone (*white arrow*). (*Courtesy of* Stephen J. Divers, Athens, GA.)

The snare is partially closed around the mesorchium, thereby isolating the testis and overlying abdominal air sac. With the snare further tightened around the mesorchium and slight lateral pressure applied to elevate the testis away from the kidney, the radio-surgery device is activated to coagulate the mesorchium and facilitate separation of the testis. The radiosurgical snare is removed and replaced by forceps that are used to retrieve the testis (**Fig. 7**). If necessary, the skin incision can be enlarged to permit the removal of a large testis. Following a final evaluation of the surgical site, the telescope is removed and both skin incisions closed routinely using single sutures. The bird then is placed into left lateral recumbency, and the procedure is repeated to remove the right testis.

Salpingohysterectomy (triple-entry technique)

To perform salpingohysterectomy, the telescope is positioned mid-way between the last rib and pubis bone, and the first cannula is placed caudal to the pubis using the same anatomic landmarks and techniques as described for orchidectomy. A second cannula is positioned immediately caudal to the last rib, at the ventral border of the flexor cruris medialis muscle, and cranial to the telescope. This second cannula is directed caudad into the left abdominal air sac using the telescope to provide direct visualization (**Fig. 8**).

Once both cannulae are positioned within the left abdominal air sac, the telescope is rotated, taking advantage of the 30° angle, to provide a caudal view of the coelom. This is achieved by supporting the telescope using gel pads or sand bags such that the light guide cable exits from the left of the telescope, and the 30° is directed caudad to image the uterus. Short Kelly dissecting forceps (3 mm) are inserted down the cranial cannula into the endoscopic field to grasp the caudal shell gland and uterus, and elevate it away from the caudal division of the kidney, ureter, vena cava, and cloaca (**Fig. 9**). A racket handle ensures that the shell gland does not slip from the jaws of the forceps during manipulation.

Short, serrated scissors (3 mm) are connected to a radiofrequency unit (initial sug-gested power setting of 5% to 8% on cut and coagulation) and inserted through the

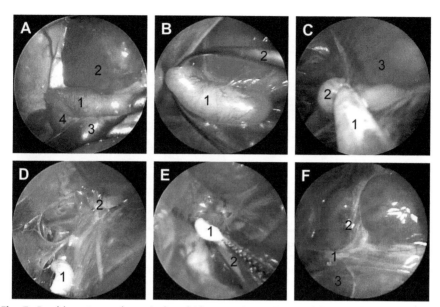

Fig. 7. Double-entry endosurgical orchidectomy in a pigeon. (*A*) View from within the cranial aspect of the left abdominal air sac demonstrating the anatomic relationship between the testis (1), cranial division of the kidney (2), vena cava (3), and adrenal gland (4). (*B*) The testis (1) is ensnared by the extended polypectomy snare (2). (*C*) The polypectomy snare (1) is retracted entrapping the testis (2) and facilitating elevation away from the cranial division of the kidney (3). (*D*) After radiosurgical activation and complete retraction of the snare, the testis (1), seen lying within the abdominal air sac, is freed from its mesorchial attachments (2) and close association with the kidney. (*E*) The testis (1) is removed from the air sac using forceps (2). (*F*) Immediate postoperative view demonstrating the coagulated remains of the mesorchium (1), mild, focal, coagulative necrosis (2) to the cranial division of the kidney, and a small defect within the abdominal air sac wall (3). (*Courtesy of* Stephen J. Divers, Athens, GA.)

caudal cannula. For right-handed surgeons, the forceps are controlled with the left hand, the scissors with the right hand, and the radiosurgery unit by foot pedal. With the reproductive tract elevated, the uterus is cut transversely close to its cloacal insertion, with the stump radiosurgically sealed. The forceps and uterus are retracted craniad to expose the ventral and dorsal ligaments of the reproductive tract. The scissors are used to cut and coagulate the ventral and dorsal ligaments and their associated blood vessels, taking care not to damage the kidney, ureter, and intestinal tract. As the dissection proceeds craniad, the telescope and light guide cable are rotated 180° to view the more cranial oviduct. The cranial aspect of the infundibulum is incised as close to the ovary as possible, but no attempt generally is made to remove the ovary because of the difficulties of maintaining hemostasis (see **Fig 9**). The cannula is slid up the shaft of the instrument to permit removal of the forceps and reproductive tract through the skin incision. Following a final inspection of the surgical site, the telescope and both cannulae are removed, and all skin incisions are closed routinely using single sutures.

Endoscopic orchidectomy and salpingohysterectomy take less than 40 minutes, and only minor complications have been reported including mild hemorrhage and focal coagulative damage to the kidney.[15] Surgical failures caused by inexperience are likely, however, unless training and practice using endoscopy trainers or cadavers

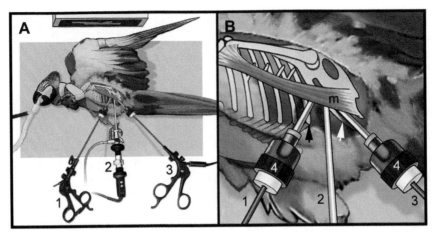

Fig. 8. (*A*) Triple-entry endosurgical salpingohysterectomy in a macaw using 3 mm forceps (1), 2.7 mm telescope with camera (2), and 3 mm scissors (3). (*B*) Close-up of the surgical site illustrating the entry of the 2.7 mm telescope (2) in front of the pubis bone (*white arrow*) at the ventral border of the flexor curis medialis muscle (m) into the abdominal air sac; insertion of the 3 mm forceps (1) behind the last rib (*black arrow*) at the ventral border of the flexor curis medialis muscle (m); and insertion of the 3 mm monopolar scissors (3) behind the pubis bone (*white arrow*) at the ventral border of the flexor cruris medialis muscle (m). The forceps and scissors are inserted through 3.5 mm plastic/graphite cannulae (4). (*Courtesy of* Stephen J. Divers, Athens, GA.)

before embarking on clinical cases. In addition, salpingohysterectomy does not appear to prevent ovarian development and ovulation, and so is unlikely to resolve hormonally derived problems in female birds. Development of an endoscopic ovariectomy technique is still required, and currently under development.

Mass resection
Double- and triple-entry techniques have been used to endoscopically debulk and remove coelomic neoplasia, abscesses, and granulomas (**Figs. 10** and **11**). In cases of bacterial or fungal infection, it is often beneficial to treat locally (by intralesional injections) and systemically to reduce the size of the abscess or granuloma before effecting endoscopic removal (see **Fig 11**). Although systems exist in human medicine to resect and remove large masses without causing contamination, this is far more difficult in the confines of the avian coelom. Therefore, the endoscopist must take precautions to remove as much material as possible and be diligent in trying not to seed infection along the instrument tracts. In addition, antimicrobial therapy should continue for several days postoperatively.

COMPLICATIONS

The major complications encountered are typically associated with anesthesia and the advanced disease state of many birds at the time of presentation. The importance of stabilization and a thorough preoperative evaluation cannot be overemphasized. Endotracheal intubation, ventilation, intravenous or intraosseous catheterization with perioperative fluid support, and warm air/water blankets are important. Most endosurgery issues are related to operator error until training and experience have been gained. The use of endoscopic radiosurgery or other hemostatic device is critical to

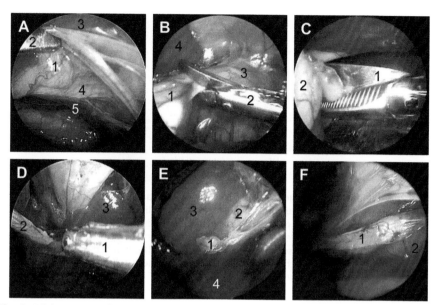

Fig. 9. Triple-entry endosurgical salpingohysterectomy in a pigeon. (*A*) View from within the caudal aspect of the left abdominal air sac. The reproductive tract (1) has been grasped with forceps (2) and elevated away from the closely associated caudal division of the kidney (3), ureter (4), and vena cava (5). (*B*) While maintaining traction on the caudal aspect of the reproductive tract (1), monopolar scissors (2) transversely incise the uterus close to its cloacal insertion (3). The caudal division of the kidney (4) is also visible. (*C*) Monopolar scissors (1) dissect the reproductive tract (2) free from its ligamentous attachments. (*D*) Dissection is continued craniad until the scissors (1) make a final transverse incision through the most proximal aspect of the oviduct (2), close to the cranial division of the kidney (3). (*E*) Postoperative view depicting a small infundibular remnant (1) and a small focal area of coagulative necrosis (2) affecting the cranial division of the kidney (3). The inactive ovary also can be seen (4) but typically is not removed. (*F*) Postoperative view of the radiosurgical-sealed uterine stump (1), adjacent to the cloaca (2). (*Courtesy of Stephen J. Divers, Athens, GA.*)

prevent serious hemorrhage. To develop an endosurgery caseload without compromising clients or patients, it is recommended that the surgeon should retain the option to convert to a traditional surgical approach if unable to perform the desired task endoscopically.

POSTOPERATIVE CARE

Birds should be supervised closely on recovery, as compromise can ensue following extubation and cessation of cardiorespiratory support. Fluid therapy and nutritional support should continue, with psittacines and passerines eating within 1 to 2 hours of recovery. Meloxicam is used routinely postoperatively, although opiates and local anesthetics could prove useful as part of a balanced approach to analgesia. Typically, birds quickly return to normal function following endosurgical procedures compared with more traditional, invasive surgery. Sutures are removed at 7 to 10 days if still present.

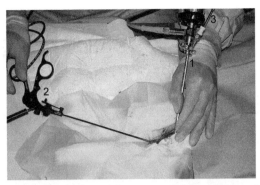

Fig. 10. Double-entry endosurgery in a cockatoo to remove an intracoelomic mass from the left abdominal air sac. The telescope (1) with camera and light guide cable attached has been inserted behind the last rib and is being triangulated with 3 mm Blakesley dissecting/biopsy forceps (2) that have been inserted just caudal to the pubis bone and into the abdominal air sac. Note the insertion of grasping forceps (3) down the operating channel of the operating sheath, which provides a second instrument (albeit dependent on the telescope). (*Courtesy of* Stephen J. Divers, Athens, GA.)

OUTCOME

The most substantial limitation to successful coelomic soft tissue surgery is the relative small size of most avian patients and the limited surgical access afforded by standard coeliotomy techniques.[16] Both of these limitations can be largely overcome by endosurgery, which provides focal magnification, illumination, and surgical access within the coelom. Each of the described techniques has advantages and disadvantages. Reports from human surgeons, however, indicate that considerable benefits may be gained from minimally invasive endosurgery.[17-22] Human laparoscopy has been credited with more rapid and accurate diagnosis, reduced need for extensive laparotomy, reduced surgical stress, improved postoperative pulmonary function, reduced hypoxemia, reduced surgical time, and faster recovery.[17,22] The disadvantage of human laparoscopy appears minimal and restricted to misdiagnosis in less than 1% of cases. No significant morbidity has been demonstrated with appropriate laparoscopic technique.[21] The efficacy, complications, and long-term effects of endosurgery have not been documented extensively in birds, although ongoing research at the University of Georgia continues to evaluate these procedures. For example, although endoscopic salpingohysterectomy prevents future egg production and dystocia, ovariectomy is required to stop reproductive physiology (including normal and abnormal behaviors and ovulation). Safe gonadectomy remains the "Holy Grail" of avian endosurgery, and remains under development.

The ability to perform endosurgery is not innate, and extensive training is undertaken by human surgeons using artificial teaching devices and supervised instruction by experienced endoscopists. Such educational tools are not readily available to the avian veterinarian, although minilaparotomy trainers can be made economically. Therefore, initial training is best achieved through participation in continuing education courses and practical laboratories. Although every opportunity should be taken to practice these techniques on animal subjects, cadavers represent a useful but imperfect model because of rapid deterioration after death. However, where this is the only available option, additional observation and assistance of an experienced endoscopist working with live birds is recommended. In those countries that permit and regulate

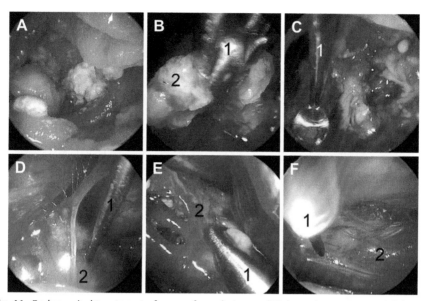

Fig. 11. Endosurgical treatment of severe fungal air sacculitis in an Amazon parrot. (*A*) View from within the left abdominal air sac demonstrating complete coverage of all viscera with *Aspergillus fumigatus*. (*B*) Single-entry endosurgical debridement using 1.7 mm biopsy forceps (1) and a 2.7 mm telescope housed within a 4.8 mm operating sheath. Large pieces of fungus (2) cannot be removed via the sheath, and the entire telescope-sheath-instrument has to be removed as a single unit. (*C*) Intralesional application of amphotericin B using a 1.7 mm remote injection needle (1) via the instrument channel of the operating sheath. (*D*) View from within the left abdominal air sac of the same bird following 15 days of antifungal therapy. The 1.7 mm remote injection needle (1) is inserted into the organizing granuloma (2), and intralesional amphotericin B administration is repeated. (*E*) The same bird following another 14 days of antifungal therapy. Double-entry endosurgery using a 2.7 mm telescope introduced behind the last rib and 3 mm Blakesley dissecting/biopsy forceps (1) introduced in front of the pubis bone. The forceps are used to remove the granuloma (2) piecemeal. (*F*) Final application of amphotericin B using the remote injection needle (1) within the abdominal air sac following granuloma removal. The kidney (2) now can be seen, and this bird continued to make a full recovery. (*Courtesy of* Stephen J. Divers, Athens, GA.)

the use of live animals for training veterinarians, nonrecovery endosurgery laboratories using anesthetized pigeons offer an unparalleled opportunity for establishing competence before embarking on clinical cases.

ACKNOWLEDGMENTS

The author is grateful to the Association of Avian Veterinarians for granting permission to reprint material that was original published in the Journal of Avian Medicine and Surgery:

Hernandez-Divers SJ. Endosurgical debridement and diode laser ablation of lung and air sac granulomas in psittacine birds. J Avian Med Surg 2002;16:138–45.

Hernandez-Divers SJ. Minimally invasive endoscopic surgery of birds. J Avian Med Surg 2005;19(2):107–20.

Hernandez-Divers SJ, et al. Endoscopic orchidectomy and salpingohysterectomy of pigeons (*Columba livia*): an avian model for minimally invasive endosurgery. J Avian Med Surg 2007;21(1):22–37.

REFERENCES

1. Cooper JE. Endoscopy in exotic species. In: Bearley MJ, Cooper JE, Sullivan M, editors. Color atlas of small animal endoscopy. St. Louis (MO): Mosby; 1991. p. 111–22.
2. Burrows CF, Heard DJ. Endoscopy in nondomestic species. In: Tams TR, editor. Small animal endoscopy. St. Louis (MO): Mosby; 1999. p. 297–321.
3. Taylor M. Endoscopic examination and biopsy techniques. In: Ritchie BW, Harrison GJ, Harrison LR, editors. Avian medicine: principles and application. Fort Worth (FL): Harrison Bird Diets International; 1994. p. 327–54.
4. Bottcher M. [Experiences with diagnostic endoscopy in birds]. Tierarztl Prax 1982;10(2):183–8 [in German].
5. Jones DM, Samour JH, Knight JA, et al. Sex determination of monomorphic birds by fibreoptic endoscopy. Vet Rec 1984;115(23):596–8.
6. Harrison GJ. Endoscopic examination of avian gonadal tissues. Vet Med Small Anim Clin 1978;73(4):479–84.
7. Ingram KA. Laparotomy technique for sex determination of psittacine birds. J Am Vet Med Assoc 1978;173(9):1244–6.
8. Hernandez-Divers SJ, Hernandez-Divers SM. Avian diagnostic endoscopy. Comp Cont Educ Pract Vet 2004;26(11):839–52.
9. Chamness CJ. Equipment for the avian and exotic endoscopist. Semin Avian Exotic Pet Med 1999;8:102–6.
10. Chamness CJ. Endoscopic instrumentation. In: Tams TR, editor. Small animal endoscopy. St. Louis (MO): Mosby; 1999. p. 1–16.
11. Hernandez-Divers SJ. Endosurgical debridement and diode laser ablation of lung and air sac granulomas in psittacine birds. J Avian Med Surg 2002;16:138–45.
12. Carpenter JW. Exotic animal formulary. 3rd edition. St Louis (MO): WB Saunders Company; 2005.
13. Pye GW, Bennett RA, Plunske R, et al. Endoscopic salpingohysterectomy of juvenile cockatiels (Nymphicus Hollandicus). J Avian Med Surg 2001;15:90–4.
14. Hernandez-Divers SJ. Minimally-invasive endoscopic surgery of birds. J Avian Med Surg 2005;19(2):107–20.
15. Hernandez-Divers SJ, Stahl SJ, Wilson GH, et al. Endoscopic orchidectomy and salpingohysterectomy of pigeons (Columba livia): an avian model for minimally invasive endosurgery. J Avian Med Surg 2007;21(1):22–37.
16. Bennett RA, Harrison GJ. Soft tissue surgery. In: Ritchie BW, Harrison GJ, Harrison LR, editors. Avian medicine: principles and application. Fort Worth (TX): Harrison Bird Diets International Incorporated; 1994. p. 1096–136.
17. Kehlet H. Surgical stress response: does endoscopic surgery confer an advantage? World J Surg 1999;23(8):801–7.
18. Corson SL, Grochmal SA. Contact laser laparoscopy has distinct advantages over alternatives. Clin Laser Mon 1990;8(1):7–9.
19. Golditch IM. Laparoscopy: advances and advantages. Fertil Steril 1971;22(5):306–10.
20. Lagares-Garcia JA, Bansidhar B, Moore RA. Benefits of laparoscopy in middle-aged patients. Surg Endosc 2003;17(1):68–72.
21. Vander Velpen GC, Shimi SM, Cuschieri A. Diagnostic yield and management benefit of laparoscopy: a prospective audit. Gut 1994;35(11):1617–21.
22. Yu SY, Chiu JH, Loong CC, et al. Diagnostic laparoscopy: indication and benefit. Zhonghua Yi Xue Za Zhi (Taipei) 1997;59(3):158–63.

Reptile Diagnostic Endoscopy and Endosurgery

Stephen J. Divers, BVetMed, DZooMed, DACZM, DipECZM(herp), FRCVS

KEYWORDS

- Reptile • Minimally invasive surgery • Endoscopy • Biopsy
- Diagnosis

The class Reptilia consists of more than 8000 species, including approximately 300 species of turtles, tortoises, and terrapins (Testudines); 2900 species of snakes (Serpentes); and 5000 species of lizards (Sauria). Only the commonly maintained companion animal species are discussed here; venomous reptiles, tuataras, and crocodilians were purposefully excluded.

There have been sporadic reports of reptile endoscopy since the 1960s. Most previous reports describe the use of endoscopy to examine or retrieve foreign objects from the gastrointestinal tract, along with descriptions of coelioscopy, bronchoscopy, and urogenital endoscopy.[1–11] More recently, further development and reviews of single- and multiple-entry techniques have expanded the applications in the Reptilia.[12–14] In particular, validation of endoscopy procedures in lizards (eg, liver and renal biopsy in iguanas), chelonians (eg, renal biopsy in various species, neonate gender identification), and snakes (eg, pulmonoscopy in royal pythons) have helped confirm safety and diagnostic value.[7,11,15] Given the often small and delicate nature of reptile pets, the continued development of minimally invasive endoscopy seems assured in these taxa.

PATIENT SELECTION

Most reptiles are presented in a state of advanced, often chronic disease, and therefore patients must be stabilized before anesthesia and surgery. The most common endoscopic procedures performed by the author include coelioscopy (lizards, chelonians), gastroscopy and cloacoscopy (all species), and tracheobronchoscopy/pulmonoscopy (all species). However, most procedures described (or necessary modifications thereof) can be undertaken in most reptiles if equipment can be matched to patient size. In addition to anesthetic complications, small patient size often presents the greatest challenge to the reptile endoscopist.

Department of Small Animal Medicine & Surgery (Zoological Medicine), College of Veterinary Medicine, University of Georgia, 501 DW Brooks Drive, Athens, GA 30602, USA
E-mail address: sdivers@uga.edu

Vet Clin Exot Anim 13 (2010) 217–242
doi:10.1016/j.cvex.2010.01.004 **vetexotic.theclinics.com**

Obesity is less of an issue, because in general reptiles store fat in discrete fat bodies rather than diffusely around organs like mammals. The benefits of endoscopy are numerous but mostly center on the fact that traditional approaches are more invasive, require longer anesthetic periods, and are associated with significantly greater procedural risks (eg, coeliotomy vs coelioscopy). In addition, the means to a definitive diagnosis relies on the demonstration of a host pathologic response (ie, histology, cytology, paired rising titres) and the causative agent (ie, microbiology, parasitology, toxicology). Given the relative paucity of serologic tests available for most reptiles combined with the 6- to 10-week delay in obtaining paired titers, the collection of tissue samples represents the most expedient means, short of necropsy, of reaching a diagnosis. The ability to examine internally and collect tissue samples has increased the array of antemortem diagnoses considerably, with accurate diagnosis resulting in more appropriate targeted therapy and improved clinical success in these otherwise stoic patients.

CONTRAINDICATIONS

Given the application of the 2.7-mm system, and more recent developments using 2- to 3-mm human pediatric equipment, the greatest limiting factor is probably the small size of most companion reptiles in combination with surgeon ability. In most cases, reptiles are chronically ill and come with inherently higher anesthetic risks. Appropriate stabilization and, in the case of endosurgery, reserving the right to delay, abort, or convert to a traditional surgical approach are important.

INSTRUMENTATION

Given the variation in reptile size and the nature of the procedures that may be performed, a variety of different endoscopes and instruments may be required (see Table 1 in the article by Stephen J. Divers elsewhere in this issue for further explanation of this topic). For most practices, the 2.7-mm system offers the greatest versatility, which can be built on as individual caseloads dictate. This system offers several advantages, including single-entry procedures, ports for air or saline infusion, and an operating channel for the introduction of 1.7-mm instruments. In addition, the 1.9-mm telescope with integrated sheath and the 1-mm semirigid miniscope are useful for smaller reptiles. For multiple-entry endoscopy, the use of 2- and 3-mm human pediatric instruments has enabled coelomic endosurgery to become a reality.[16]

PATIENT EVALUATION

Knowledge of species-specific anatomy, physiology, husbandry, and nutritional requirements are vital to properly evaluate the management and medical history of a reptile. Inexperienced clinicians are directed to reviews on the subject and should prepare ahead of time.[17,18] Complete physical examination, including accurate body weight, is essential, but may require sedation or anesthesia for aggressive snakes or uncooperative animals, particularly chelonians. Serial clinicopathologic data can be helpful to quantify dehydration, indicate infection/inflammation, and indicate potential organ damage or dysfunction. However, most published reference ranges are too broad to be valuable unless patient data are severely abnormal. Complete blood counts and biochemistry panels are recommended, and even in animals less than 100 g, hematocrit and total solids can still be obtained.

PATIENT PREPARATION

In most cases, sick reptiles present with anorexia lasting days to months, and fasting is usually not a concern. However, when dealing with animals that are still feeding, fasting should be in accordance with body size and feeding strategy. For example, a 20-kg python would typically be fasted for 3 to 4 weeks, whereas a 500-g cornsnake would require only 5 to 7 days. Likewise, fasting a carnivorous turtle for 2 to 3 days would reduce the volume of food in the stomach, whereas fasting an herbivorous tortoise for the same period would have little effect given that most ingesta is located within the large intestine. As a general guide, a single feeding cycle should be avoided before anesthesia and surgery.

In general, fluid therapy is the mainstay of stabilization, and rehydration using crystalloid fluids (with an osmolarity of 260–290 mOsm/L) at 25 to 45 mL/kg per day is recommended.[19] Fluids may be given intravenously or intraosseously for critical cases, or intracoelomically, subcutaneously, or orally. Avoiding oral or intracoelomic fluids immediately before gastroscopy or coelioscopy is advisable.

ANESTHESIA AND MONITORING

Certain examinations (eg, stomatoscopy, cloacoscopy) may be possible in the conscious or sedated patient using a mouth gag and appropriate restraint, but complete immobilization is preferred to avoid risking damage to equipment, patient, or staff. General anesthesia is recommended for all endoscopy procedures (including oral and cloacal examinations) and is required for any invasive procedures (including coelioscopy).[9,20] Conscious coelioscopic examinations may be acceptable in research or free-ranging wildlife investigations under an appropriate experimental license, but for clinical medicine analgesia and anesthesia must be provided. Although some authors have reported using only local anesthesia for chelonian coelioscopy, this likely provides inadequate analgesia for more involved coelioscopic procedures.[21] In a recent comparison of local versus general anesthesia for chelonian coelioscopy, objective anesthetic scores were significantly better for procedures conducted with general anesthesia than with local lidocaine alone.[9]

Particular regard should be given to maintenance of an appropriate temperature within the upper range of the species-specific preferred temperature zone (often 25–30°C, 77–86°F). For small lizards and snakes (<200 g), the author prefers to induce anesthesia in an induction chamber (eg, Ziplock bag) using 5% isoflurane or 8% sevoflurane, intubated, and maintained on isoflurane or sevoflurane. Larger lizards, snakes, and chelonians (>200 g) the author typically induces using intravenous propofol (3–10 mg/kg), intubates, and maintains on isoflurane or sevoflurane.

When intubation and gas anesthesia is either impractical or unavailable, a combination of ketamine (10 mg/kg), medetomidine (0.1 mg/kg), and morphine (1.5 mg/kg) given by single intramuscular or intravenous injection is effective. This combination has proven sufficient for coelioscopy in numerous chelonian species, particularly hatchlings and small juveniles, and is often augmented with buffered lidocaine at the surgical site (**Fig. 1**). Reversal using naloxone (0.2 mg/kg) and atipamezole (0.5 mg/kg) seems rapid and complete.

Uncuffed endotracheal tubes are used for chelonians, smaller snakes, and lizards. Cuffed tubes can be used for larger squamates.

All reptiles become apneic at surgical anesthetic planes, and therefore ventilation (typically 1–6 breaths per minute) is required for prolonged procedures, and should be modified to maintain end-tidal capnography readings of 15 to 25 mmHg. Intraoperative vascular access can be achieved using intraosseous or intravenous catheters.

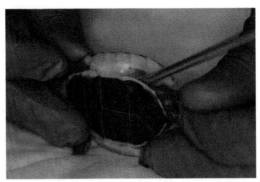

Fig. 1. Performing coelioscopy for gender identification in a 10-g hatchling turtle under general anesthesia using a triple injectable combination of ketamine, medetomidine, and morphine. (*Courtesy of* Stephen J. Divers, Athens, GA.)

Caudal (ventral tail) intravenous catheters are preferred for lizards and snakes, and (following a surgical cut-down procedure) jugular catheters for chelonians. Intraoperative fluid rates of 3 mL/kg are adequate. Anesthesia should be monitored by evaluating withdrawal reflexes, Doppler, pulse oximetry, and end-tidal capnography. In general pulse rates should not decrease more than 50% from conscious baseline levels. Preventing end-tidal capnography values from dropping below 15 mmHg through excessive ventilation seems to speed the return to spontaneous breathing on recovery. Reptiles should be monitored regularly even after extubation, because some may regress into unconsciousness and apnea.

Controversy remains over the use of opiate analgesics in reptiles, and taxa-specific effects have been documented; however, morphine (1.5 mg/kg) seems effective for chelonians, whereas very high doses of morphine or butorphanol seem to be required for some lizards and snakes.[22,23] Meloxicam (0.2 mg/kg) is used routinely for all species, and may be repeated after 48 to 72 hours if necessary.[24]

DIAGNOSTIC PROCEDURES

The general techniques for reptile endoscopy are similar to those used for domesticated animals. However, the fact that most pet reptiles weigh less than 1 kg requires careful control, with the base of the telescope, eyepiece, and camera supported using the superior hand and the terminal end held by thumb and forefinger of the inferior hand. Handling the telescope in this fashion provides fine control without tremor.

Tracheoscopy and Pulmonoscopy

Depending on the size of the reptile, a 2.7-mm, 1.9-mm, or 1.0-mm endoscope can be used to examine the glottis and trachea of most lizards, chelonians, and snakes (**Fig. 2**).[12] Using a protection sheath with the finer telescopes is always preferable, but the increased diameter may be prohibitive. Rigid scopes of sufficient length can usually be directed into the lungs of lizards by carefully manipulating the lizard's head, neck, and body. For large snakes and chelonians, fine-diameter flexible endoscopes or video-bronchoscopes will permit deeper examination into the lungs.[25,26]

The reptile is positioned in dorsal or sternal recumbency, with head and neck extended. A mouth gag is recommended to guard against a lightly anesthetized reptile from biting down on the endoscope. The endoscope should be inserted through the glottis and gently advanced under direct visual control to avoid damaging the mucosa.

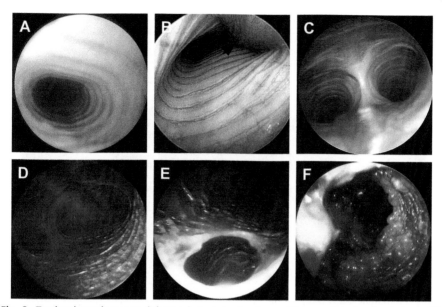

Fig. 2. Tracheobronchoscopy. (*A*) Greek tortoise trachea with complete tracheal rings. (*B*) Royal python trachea with obvious dorsal ligament (*arrow*). (*C*) Tracheal bifurcation and primary bronchi in a green iguana. (*D*) Simple sac-like lung in a green iguana. (*E*) Compartmentalized lung in a panther chameleon. (*F*) Granulomatous pneumonia from *Mycobacterium* spp in a ball python. (*Courtesy of* Stephen J. Divers, Athens, GA.)

Complete tracheal occlusion for several minutes is well tolerated by anesthetized reptiles, and an alternative airway is not necessary.

A tracheal approach to the chelonian lung is particularly difficult because of the narrow trachea and meandering primary bronchi. It is possible in the largest species (eg, giant tortoises and sea turtles) using fine flexible endoscopes, but not in smaller specimens, and therefore two alternative approaches to the chelonian lung have been developed.[12] The first requires a 4-mm temporary osteotomy in the carapace over the suspected lesion, pinpointed by diagnostic imaging. The pleuropulmonary membrane is punctured using a trocar or straight hemostats while the animal is held at maximal inspiration. Leakage of anesthetic gases confirms entry into the lung, and additional anesthetic gas scavenging should be positioned close to the surgical site. The sheathed telescope can then be inserted into the lung for examination (**Fig. 3**). The osteotomy can be temporarily maintained with a catheter and injection cap secured within the hole to permit intrapulmonic therapy. Alternatively, the osteotomy can be closed using an epoxy or acrylic compound. The shell heals within 12 weeks.

A second method for chelonians involves a prefemoral approach to the lung. This method is most suitable for species with a relatively large prefemoral fossa that can facilitate surgical entry into the coelom with identification of the caudoventral lung. A small (1–2 cm) craniocaudal incision is made in the craniodorsal aspect of the prefemoral fossa (**Fig. 4**A). The coelomic membrane may need to be perforated and opened using hemostats in order to identify the lung (aided by frequent ventilation). Two stay sutures are placed through the caudoventral border of the lung to elevate the pulmonary tissue lung to the level of the skin incision. A stab incision through a thin and relatively avascular portion of the exposed lung provides access for the

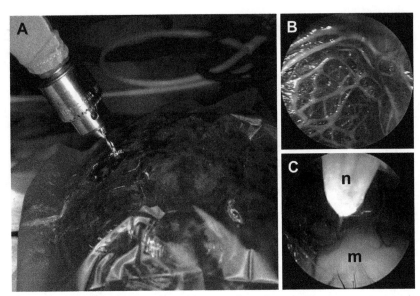

Fig. 3. Chelonian transcarapacial pulmonoscopy. (*A*) Drilling a 4-mm temporary osteotomy through the carapace of a Greek tortoise to access the lung. (*B*) Normal view of the chelonian lung through the temporary osteotomy. (*C*) Large mass (m) within the lung of a juvenile loggerhead sea turtle through a temporary carapacial osteotomy. Aspiration is first attempted using an endoscopic needle (n) and, if not fluid-filled, biopsies are taken. In this case the lesion was an encapsulated fungal granuloma. (*Courtesy of* Stephen J. Divers, Athens, GA.)

telescope. The pulmonary examination can then proceed from caudal to cranial, and in some species it is possible to move cranial to the opening of the primary bronchus (**Fig. 4**B, C). On withdrawal, the lung must be closed using fine suture material to avoid postoperative pneumocoelom and/or subcutaneous emphasema.

A transcutaneous approach to the lung of snakes has also been described.[11,27] This technique involves a mini-coeliotomy approach to the lung approximately 35% to 45% from snout-to-vent, on the right side (or either left or right side for boas and pythons because they have two lungs). After a 1-cm skin incision and blunt dissection through an intercostal space, the lung is identified as it is inflated, grasped, secured, and punctured using a scalpel blade before insertion of the telescope. Depending on the size of the snake and telescope, this approach enables evaluation of the distal trachea, primary and intrapulmonary bronchus, cranial faveolar lung, transitional zone, and the caudal air sac (**Fig. 5**). The lung and skin are closed routinely using single sutures.

Biopsies can be readily collected from within the pulmonary system, and a study in snakes showed that 1.7-mm biopsies can be safely collected without deleterious effects.[11] These biopsies can be submitted for histopathology, microbiology, and parasitology. In general, gently shaking the lung biopsy free into a small volume of saline before transferring to 10% neutral buffered formalin reduces artifacts.

Stomatoscopy and Gastroscopy

Sternal or dorsal recumbency with head and neck extended is preferred for stomatoscopy and gastroscopy. Positioning the reptile close to the table edge or raised above the table surface is often helpful. The rigid telescope-sheath system can be used to examine the buccal cavity, esophagus, and stomach of small lizards and chelonians (**Fig. 6**). Flexible endoscopes are required to gain access to the stomach for most

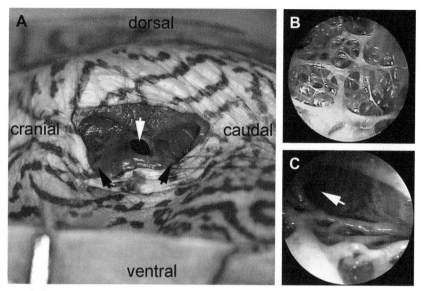

Fig. 4. Chelonian transcutaneous, prefemoral pulmonoscopy. (*A*) Surgical view of the prefemoral fossa of a map turtle after a mini-coeliotomy incision. Two fine stay sutures (*black arrows*) have been placed to elevate the lung to the skin incision, and a small stab incision has been made through an avascular window (*white arrow*) into the lung. (*B*) Endoscopic view from within the lung of a map turtle (*Graptemys*) showing the characteristic faveolar to edicular nature of the tissue. (*C*) Endoscopic view from within the lung of Greek tortoise (*Testudo*) showing the opening to the primary bronchus (*arrow*). (*Courtesy of* Stephen J. Divers, Athens, GA.)

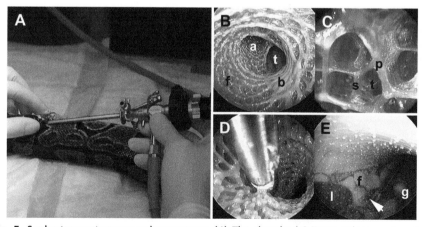

Fig. 5. Snake transcutaneous pulmonoscopy. (*A*) The sheathed 2.7-mm telescope inserted through the lateral body wall and introduced into the cranial lung of a research ball python that has not been draped to permit visualization of the snake's position and surgical entry site. (*B*) Cranial view of the python lung showing the distal trachea (t), intrapulmonary bronchus (b), anterior lung lobe (a), and the faveolar lung tissue (f). (*C*) Close-up view of the faveolar region showing the primary (p), secondary (s), and tertiary (t) septae of the anterior vascular lung. (*D*) Lung biopsy using the 1.7-mm biopsy forceps. (*E*) View of the thin, transparent, caudal airsac through which the caudal edge of the liver (l), fat body (f), gastrointestinal tract (g), and caudal vena cava (*arrow*) can be seen. (*Courtesy of* Stephen J. Divers, Athens, GA.)

snakes and larger reptiles of other orders (**Fig. 7**). Air insufflation can be used to dilate the tract, providing good exposure for detecting gross lesions and foreign bodies. Warm saline irrigation provides superior clarity, especially when examining for mucosal detail, although tracheal intubation is essential to avoid aspiration. Whether air or saline is used, gently dilating the tract as the endoscope is advanced is important to avoid damage and laceration to the wall. Foreign bodies can be readily retrieved, and biopsy collection should be undertaken with care to avoid perforation of the intestinal tract, which is more likely in the thin-walled esophagus than the stomach.

Cloacoscopy

Although snakes can also be positioned in sternal or dorsal recumbency, chelonians and lizards are easier in dorsal. Rigid endoscopy using warm saline irrigation promotes unparalleled examination of the proctodeum, urodeum, and coprodeum (**Fig. 8**) and detailed appraisal of the distal colon, cloacal mucosa, urogenital papillae, oviductal openings in females, and (when present) the urethral opening and bladder. With practice, the endoscope can be directed through the urethra into the thin-walled bladder in chelonians and some lizards, and through the distal oviducts of reproductively active females. Cloacoscopy has been used to remove shell and egg material from the distal oviducts, and as a guide for the exteriorization of partially prolapsed tissue and resection. Mucosal biopsies should be conducted carefully, especially from the colon because of its thin nature and the risk for perforation.

More detailed information on the use of endoscopy for evaluation and surgery of the reproductive tract is provided by Innis elsewhere in this issue.

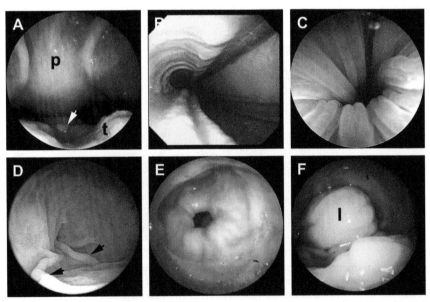

Fig. 6. Stomatoscopy, esophagoscopy and gastroscopy. (*A*) Oral cavity of a radiated tortoise showing the choana and palate (p), fleshy tongue (t), and glottis (*arrow*). (*B*) Air-distended esophagus of a burmese python. (*C*) Saline-infusion view of the green iguana esophagus. (*D*) Stomach of a savannah monitor lizard with normal rugal folds (*arrows*). (*E*) Gastric hypertrophy in a corn snake with cryptosporidiosis. (*F*) Leiomyoma (l) obstructing the pyloric outflow in a colubrid snake that presented with chronic regurgitation. (*Courtesy of* Stephen J. Divers, Athens, GA.)

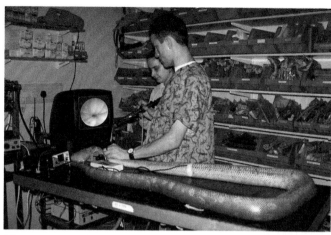

Fig. 7. Flexible gastroscopy in a color-mutant burmese python. (*Courtesy of* Stephen J. Divers, Athens, GA.)

Coelioscopy

Because reptiles lack a true abdomen, the term *coelioscopy* is preferred over *laparoscopy*. For a detailed discussion of generic laparoscopy methodologies, readers are referred to the dedicated literature, because this article only highlights reptile specifics.[28–31] Laparoscopy has been shown to offer significant advantages over traditional surgical options, both in human and veterinary medicine. In particular,

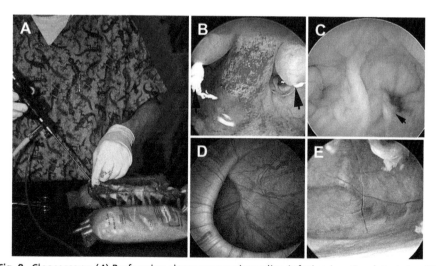

Fig. 8. Cloacoscopy. (*A*) Performing cloacoscopy using saline infusion in a Greek tortoise. (*B*) View within the urodeum of a green iguana with uric acid emerging from the urogenital papillae (*arrows*). (*Courtesy of* Dr Scott Stahl, DVM, DABVP(avian), Fairfax, VA.) (*C*) Urodeum and oviductal openings of a Hognose snake that presented with nonspecific signs. Note the discharge emanating from one of the oviducts (*arrow*) that was associated with retained egg material. (*Courtesy of* Dr Scott Stahl, DVM, DABVP(avian), Fairfax, VA.) (*D*) Distal colon of a royal python showing normal spiral folds. (*E*) View from within the bladder of a green iguana. (*Courtesy of* Stephen J. Divers, Athens, GA.)

laparoscopy is, with practice, faster, less traumatic, and associated with less postoperative pain, and provides a more rapid return to normal function.[32–43] Until the advent of 2- and 3-mm human pediatric equipment, laparoscopy was limited to a single-entry system using the sheathed telescope; however, multiple-entry techniques are now possible and practical for animals larger than 500 g.[44]

Precise positioning for coelioscopy depends on the reptile's body shape and conformation, the structures of interest, and the preferences of the endoscopist.[13] The entry site is aseptically prepared and draped, and adhesive clear plastic drapes permit better visualization of the patient. Insufflation is essential for lizards and snakes and, although the shell prevents coelomic collapse, can still be helpful in chelonians in some situations. Typically carbon dioxide insufflation pressures of 3 to 5 mmHg are used, which are lower than those recommended for mammals (8–14 mmHg). In some situations, saline infusion may be preferred over gas. In the author's experience, this is especially true when dealing with hatchlings and other very small reptiles, or when dealing with aquatic animals, in which residual gas may have a negative effect on postoperative buoyancy.

Lizards

Dorsoventrad compressed lizards (eg, bearded dragons) are positioned in dorsal recumbency, whereas laterally compressed lizards (eg, chameleons) are best placed in lateral. Round-bodied lizards (eg, green iguanas) can be positioned in either lateral or dorsal recumbency, but lateral is generally preferred and allows access to more structures. Given the relatively small size of most pet lizards, a single paramedian or paralumbar entry point usually permits examination of most, if not all, of the coelomic structures (**Fig. 9**). Although anatomic differences exist among families, the green iguana is a useful model for saurian coelioscopy.[45] In the iguana, visualization of lung, liver, pancreas, small intestine, large intestine, ovary, oviduct, testis, epididymis, vas deferens, bladder, fat body, or kidney is not significantly different for the left and right approaches. However, a left lateral approach to the heart, stomach, and spleen and a right lateral approach to the gall bladder are preferred. Right-handed surgeons will find that a left paralumbar approach is preferable, unless physical examination or diagnostic imaging dictate a right-sided problem.

The iguana is positioned in lateral recumbency, with the left pelvic limb taped caudad against the tail base. The entry area is bordered craniad by the ribs, dorsad by the spine, and caudad by the pelvic limb (see **Fig. 9**). Aseptically, a small skin incision is made in the center of the defined area. The skin and underlying muscle are grasped and elevated away from the coelomic viscera, and small haemostats are gently forced through the coelomic musculature and into the coelomic cavity. It is wise to temporarily cease artificial ventilation until the telescope has been introduced into the coelom, thereby reducing the possibility of damage to an inflated lung. The hemostats are removed and replaced by the sheath and obturator (with insufflation line attached to one of the ports). By making a small skin incision and breach in the muscle, the sheath will be tight-fitting and insufflation gas leakage will be minimal. Once in place, the obturator is removed and replaced with the telescope. Once insufflated the tip of the telescope may need to be touched against a coelomic membrane to clean the terminal lens of condensation or tissue fluid. If fat or blood is on the lens, often the telescope will need to be removed from the sheath, cleaned with gauze moistened with sterile saline, and replaced.

On entry through a left paralumbar approach in the lizard, the first organ to note is the large brown liver lying in the mid-ventral coelom (**Fig. 10**A). Advancing the scope craniad will reveal the heart at the cranioventral extent of the coelom, close to the

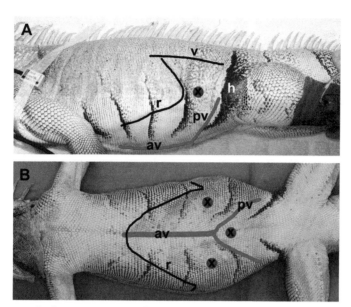

Fig. 9. Suggested telescope entry sites for coelioscopy in lizards. (*A*) For a lateral entry into the coelom, the entry point (x) is bordered craniad by the last rib (r), dorsad by the lateral processes of the lumbar vertebrae (v), caudad by the musculature of the hindlimb (h), and ventrad by the ventral abdominal (av) and pelvic veins (pv). (*B*) For a ventral approach to the coelom, insertion points (x) may be in the midline, behind the anastomoses of the lateral pelvic veins (pv), or lateral to the ventral abdominal vein (av), caudal to the last rib (r), and cranial to the pelvic veins (pv). (*Courtesy of* Stephen J. Divers, Athens, GA.)

coelomic inlet (**Fig. 10**B). Iguanas have no diaphragmatic, postpulmonary, or longitudinal membranes. These membranes do exist to a greater or lesser extent in tegus and monitors (**Fig. 10**C). Minor perforation of these membranes by the telescope will not cause harm, but care is required to avoid perforating viscera, or damaging the more caudad heart.

Dorsal to the heart and extending to mid-coelom are the paired lungs (**Fig. 10**D). Lung ventilation will be substantially reduced during carbon dioxide insufflation, and careful communication with the anesthetist is required to balance inspiration and coelomic pressures. Caudal to the lungs, in the mid-coelom, is the stomach with the spleen—an elongated dark red organ in iguanas—situated close behind (**Fig. 10**E). Careful examination medial to the stomach and spleen will reveal the splenic limb of the pancreas. The gonads are located just caudal to the spleen, either side of dorsal midline.

Rigid endoscopy can be used to determine the gender of reptiles, even at a very early age. This technique is extremely useful in monomorphic species, or in an endangered species breeding program to determine gender in neonates or juveniles.[9] Endoscopy also provides feedback on reproductive activity and disease. The testis is usually ovoid and smooth, and size may vary dramatically with season (see **Fig. 10**E). The immature or inactive ovary appears as a cluster of small, fluid-filled follicles (**Fig. 10**F). As the ovary matures, some of the follicles will enlarge and appear yellow to orange in color as they fill with yolk. Some species of lizards (eg, tegus, monitors) have thin posthepatic or postpulmonary membranes that may be pigmented and obscure the gonads. For better visualization, the membrane can be breached through

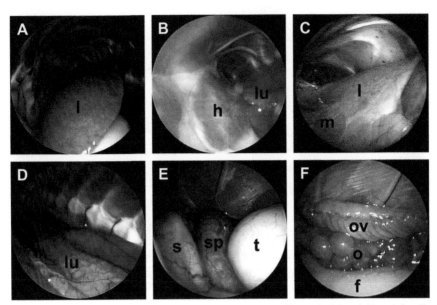

Fig. 10. Lizard coelioscopy (left lateral approach, CO_2 insufflation). (*A*) Left liver lobe (l) of an iguana. (*B*) Heart (h) and lung (lu) of a green iguana. Note the absence of a post-pulmonary membrane. (*C*) Left liver lobe (l) behind the posthepatic membrane (m) of a monitor lizard. (*D*) Lung (lu) of an iguana. Note the absence of a postpulmonary membrane in this species. (*E*) Stomach (s), spleen (sp), and testis (t) of a male green iguana. (*F*) Oviduct (ov), ovary (o), and fat body (f) in a female green iguana. (*Courtesy of* Stephen J. Divers, Athens, GA.)

grasping and tearing with retrieval forceps, or incising using scissors. Care must be taken not to damage the follicles, because leakage results in coelomitis.

Dorsal to the gonads are the adrenal glands lying adjacent to the renal veins (**Fig. 11**A). The vas deferens of males and oviducts of females are also visible and can be followed caudad to the pelvic inlet. The kidneys of most lizards are situated in the caudodorsal coelom; however, those of the iguana are intrapelvic but can still be visualized (**Fig. 11**B). Moving ventrad from the pelvic inlet, the bladder (if present) and fat body can be seen (**Fig. 11**C). A left paralumbar approach will reveal the small intestine and terminal colon; however, a right paralumbar approach will provide access to the gall bladder and, in iguanas and other herbivorous lizards a large cecum (**Fig. 11**D). Most of the pancreas is easier to locate through a right approach, residing caudal to the liver and gall bladder and closely associated with the duodenum (**Fig. 11**E). On the right side, the heart is partially obscured by the ascending vena cava (**Fig. 11**F).

Snakes

Snakes are less commonly subjected to coelomic endoscopy because (1) they have more diffuse coelomic fat, (2) all major organs cannot be examined through a single entry point, and (3) insufflation is generally more difficult. Nonetheless, if a targeted endoscopic approach to a single coelomic region is required, lateral entry between the ribs in larger snakes and ventrolateral entry just medial to the ribs in smaller snakes are practical (**Fig. 12**A).[13] A recently developed technique for liver biopsy entails

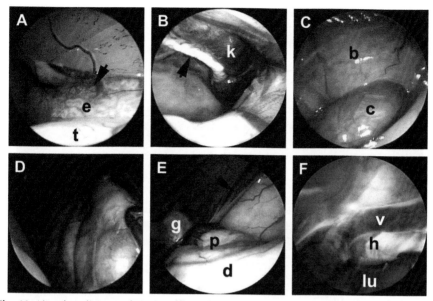

Fig. 11. Lizard coelioscopy (CO_2 insufflation). (*A*) Epididymis (e) and adrenal gland (*arrow*) lying dorsal to the testis (t) in a male iguana (left lateral approach). (*B*) Normal vas deferens (*arrow*) and kidney (k) emerging from the pelvic inlet in a green iguana (left lateral approach). (*C*) Bladder (b) and distal colon (c) in a green iguana (left lateral approach). (*D*) Loops of small bowel in a green iguana (left lateral approach). (*E*) Gall bladder (g), pancreas (p), duodenum (d), and ventral abdominal vein (*arrow*) in a green iguana (right lateral approach). (F) Cranial lung (lu) and caudal vena cava (v), partially obscuring the heart (*h*) in a green iguana (right lateral approach). (*Courtesy of* Stephen J. Divers, Athens, GA.)

access through the pulmonoscopy approach to the serpentine airsac. From within the airsac, the liver can be visualized and biopsied (**Fig. 12**B–D).

Chelonians

With the chelonian supported in lateral recumbency, the most useful coelioscopic approach is through the left or right prefemoral fossa (**Fig. 13**).[13] Right-handed surgeons will generally find it easier to enter the left prefemoral fossa, and left-handed surgeons the right. In general, unless diagnostic imaging dictates a unilateral problem, the surgeon's preference can prevail. A large bladder can hinder coelioscopy, and chelonians should be encouraged to urinate before surgery, which can be achieved through bathing the animal or gentle digital manipulation of the cloaca before anesthetic induction.

The pelvic limb is retracted and taped caudad to expose the prefemoral fossa. In chelonians with a well-developed plastron hinge (eg, box turtles) placing a wedge between the caudal plastron and carapace is wise to maintain exposure. After aseptic preparation, a small (2–4 mm) craniocaudal skin incision is made in the center of the prefemoral fossa. The subcutaneous fat and connective tissues are bluntly dissected using hemostats down to the coelomic aponeurosis (formed by the broad tendinous portions of the transverse and oblique abdominal muscles) being careful to remain cranial to the sartorius muscle and ventral to the iliacus muscle that lies between the femur and ventral surface of the ilium. The coelomic aponeurosis is penetrated through advancing hemostats (or the sheath and obturator) toward the head. Some

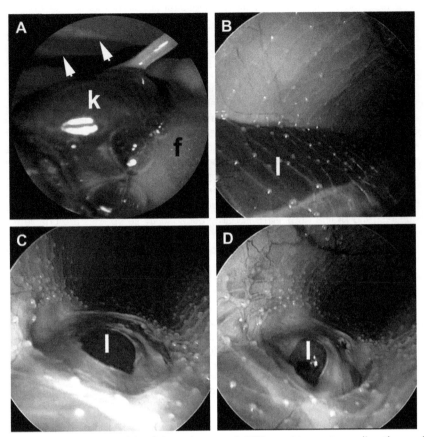

Fig. 12. Snake coelioscopy. (*A*) Left lateral approach 82% snout-to-vent revealing the caudal pole of the left kidney (k), fat body (f), and ribs (*arrows*) in a boa constrictor. (*B*) Ball python liver (l) viewed from within the airsac of the right lung. (*C*) The airsac and serosal membranes have been incised to expose the liver parenchyma (l). (*D*) View of the liver (l) after biopsy using 1.7-mm forceps. (*Courtesy of* Stephen J. Divers, Athens, GA.)

force is required to breach the coleomic membrane and gain access to the coelomic cavity (**Fig. 14**).

The dark red-brown liver is the most obvious organ to use for orientation (**Fig. 15A**). The heart is cranioventral to the liver and partially obscured by a prominent pericardium (**Fig. 15B**). The stomach is most prominent on the left (**Fig. 15C**) and, although potentially seen from either lateral, the pancreas and closely associated duodenum are easier to see from the right (**Fig. 15D**). The gall bladder is obvious and associated with the caudal edge of the right liver lobe (**Fig. 15E**), but the spleen is often hard to locate under the right liver lobe, close to the duodenum and pancreas (**Fig. 15F**).

The ventral aspects of the lungs are located dorsad, and are most obvious in species that lack a prominent postpulmonary membrane (**Fig. 16A**). The colon, gonads, oviducts (in females), bladder, and kidneys can be viewed from either side. The bladder is situated in the most dependent area, whereas the ovaries and oviducts of reproductively active females can occupy much of the coelom (**Fig. 16B, C**). The male testes (cream, yellow, or brown in color) are situated in the caudodorsal coelom and closely associated with the vasa deferentia,

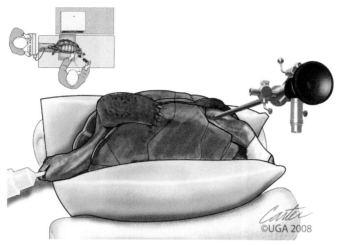

Fig. 13. Operating room layout and positioning for a left prefemoral approach in front of the pelvic limb to access the chelonian coelomic cavity. (*Courtesy of* Stephen J. Divers, Athens, GA.)

epididymides, adrenal glands, and retrocoelomic kidneys (**Fig. 16**D). Recently, endoscopy was shown to accurately identifies gender in hatchling and neonate chelonians as small as 10 g (**Fig. 16**E, F).[9] More detailed information on the use of endoscopy for evaluation and surgery of the reproductive tract is provided by Innis elsewhere in this issue.

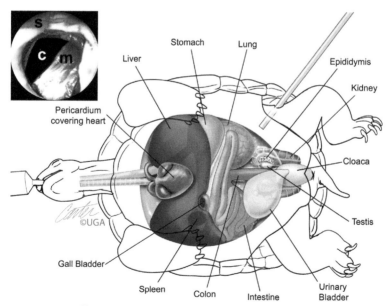

Fig. 14. Diagram to illustrate position and orientation of coelomic viscera inside a male chelonian. Note the entry position of the telescope through the prefemoral fossa and the asymmetry of certain organs. (*Insert*) View through the skin incision (s), showing the coelomic membrane (m) and penetration into the coelom (c). (*Courtesy of* Stephen J. Divers, Athens, GA.)

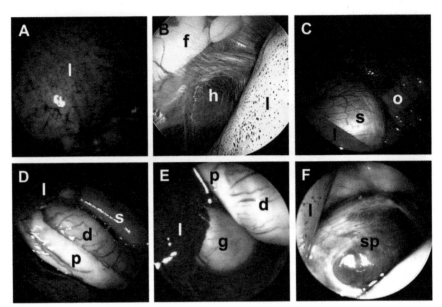

Fig. 15. Chelonian coelioscopy (CO_2 insufflation). (*A*) Normal liver (l) in a radiated tortoise (left prefemoral approach). (*B*) Heart (h) and pericardial fat (f) behind the coelomic membrane of a yellow-bellied slider. Note the pale liver (l) within the coelomic cavity (left prefemoral approach). (*C*) Stomach (s), liver (l), and oviduct (o) in a red-foot tortoise (left prefemoral approach). (*D*) Liver (l), pancreas (p) with closely associated duodenum (d), and stomach (s) in a red-eared slider (left prefemoral approach). (*E*) Pancreas (p), duodenum (d), and gall bladder (g) embedded within the caudal aspect of the right liver lobe (l) in a red-eared slider (right prefemoral approach). (*F*) Spleen (sp) lying under the right liver lobe (l) in a yellow-bellied slider (right prefemoral approach). (*Courtesy of* Stephen J. Divers, Athens, GA.)

The kidneys are retrocoelomic, residing behind an often transparent coelomic membrane (**Fig. 17**A). When presented with a pigmented coelomic membrane, the close association with the testis (or immature ovary) can help indicate their location (**Fig. 17**B). However, in adult females in which the ovary and suspensory ligament have enlarged and fallen away from the pigmented coelomic membrane, locating the kidneys can be challenging unless they are grossly abnormal (**Fig. 17**C).[15] An extracoelomic approach to the chelonian kidney is possible in species with a more flattened carapace, and does not require entry into the coelomic cavity. The sheathed endoscope is gently advanced from the same prefemoral skin incision in a caudodorsal direction between the coelomic aponeurosis and the broad iliacus muscle. A combination of gentle lateral movements of the telescope tip and intermittent insufflation are used to further separate the coelomic aponeurosis from the adjacent musculature to reveal the kidneys (**Fig. 17**D).

PATHOLOGY AND ENDOSCOPIC BIOPSY

In reptiles, various pathologies may be appreciated endoscopically, often with surprisingly few clinicopathologic or discernible radiographic or ultrasonographic changes (**Fig. 18**A–E). Tissue samples can be easily harvested from most organs and generally

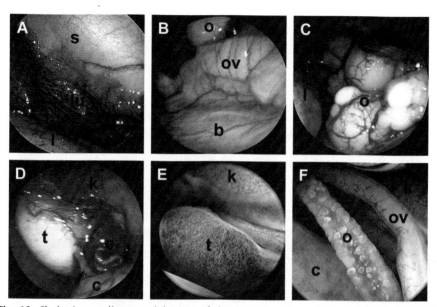

Fig. 16. Chelonian coelioscopy. (*A*) View of the serosal surface of the dorsal shell (s), left lung (lu), and liver (l) in a red-eared slider (left prefemoral approach, CO_2 insufflation). (*B*) Urinary bladder (b), oviduct (ov), and ovary (o) in an African spurred tortoise (left prefemoral approach, CO_2 insufflation). (*C*) Mature ovary (o) extending to the caudal edge of the left liver lobe (l) in a Hermann's tortoise (left prefemoral approach, air insufflation). (*D*) Testis (t), epididymis (e), and vas deferens (*arrow*) in the caudodorsal coelom of a red-eared slider. Note the closely associated retrocoelomic kidney (k) and the distal colon (c) (left prefemoral approach, air insufflation). (*E*) Immature testis (t) closely associated with the kidney (k) in a hatchling Chinese box turtle (left prefemoral approach, saline infusion). (*F*) Immature ovary (o) and oviduct (ov) closely associated with the kidney (k) and distal colon (c) in a hatchling Chinese box turtle (left prefemoral approach, saline infusion). (*Courtesy of Stephen J. Divers, Athens, GA.*)

any abnormal soft tissue structure. Liver disease may be focal or diffuse, and although the caudal edge is easiest to sample, biopsies can also be taken from the surface by first incising the serosal covering (**Fig. 18F**). Various renal diseases have also been described (**Fig. 19A, B**).[15,46] In lizards and snakes, the lobulated kidney is easy to approach and biopsy directly (**Fig. 19C**). However, in chelonians, its flattened retrocoelomic position first requires incision of the coelomic membrane if accessed using a coelioscopic approach (**Fig. 19D–F**).

SURGICAL PROCEDURES

An endoscope-assisted procedure is a hybrid that combines elements of endoscopy with traditional surgery. An assortment of endoscope-assisted coelomic procedures, including enterotomy, enterectomy, cystotomy, oophorectomy, salpingotomy, and salpingohysterectomy, are now possible. Of particular note is chelonian ovariectomy or oophorectomy, in which the endoscope is used to identify and guide the exteriorization of the ovaries with surgical resection completed outside the coelom.[14] Many of the endosurgical techniques that have been developed in chelonians center around

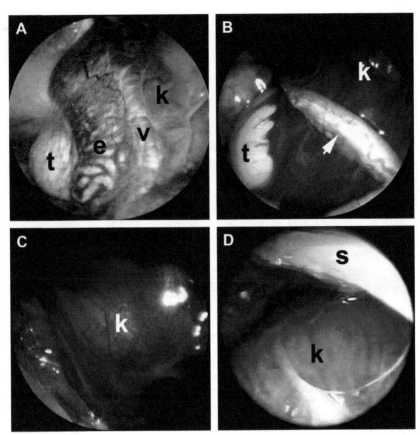

Fig. 17. Chelonian renal examination (left prefemoral approach, CO_2 insufflation). (*A*) View of the retrocoelomic kidney (k), renal vasculature (v), and closely associated testis (t) and epididymis (e) in a male red-eared slider. Note that renal visualization is possible because of the transparent nature of the coelomic membrane. (*B*) View of the same caudodorsal region in an adult male Greek tortoise. The retrocoelomic kidney (k) is obscured by the pigmented coelomic membrane; however, its position can be determined by the obvious testis (t) and vas deferens (*arrow*). (*C*) View of the same caudodorsal region in an adult female Greek tortoise with the retrocoelomic kidney (k) obscured by a pigmented membrane. With no closely associated gonad to indicate the kidney's location, the endoscopist must rely on accurate anatomic knowledge alone. (*D*) Direct, extracoelomic view of the kidney (k) and internal surface of the caudodorsal carapace (s) in a loggerhead sea turtle. (*Courtesy of* Stephen J. Divers, Athens, GA.)

their reproductive tract, and more detailed information is provided by Innis elsewhere in this issue.

Advances in reptile endosurgery, and specifically multiple-entry techniques, have been made possible by expanding the single-entry technique into a multiple-entry system using 2-, 3-, and 5-mm human laparoscopy instruments. Orchidectomy, oophorectomy, and mass/cyst resection have become possible in lizards and more recently in chelonians. Cannulae positioning and instrument entry sites are dependent on the objectives of surgery and the regional anatomy of the patient.

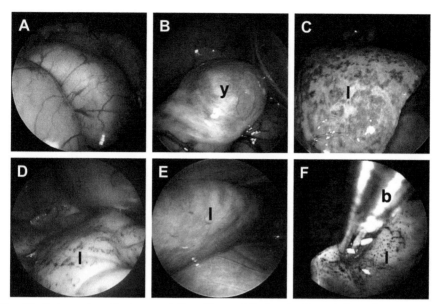

Fig. 18. Endoscopic pathology and liver biopsy. (*A*) Grossly distended small intestine in a Russian tortoise. This herbivorous tortoise was fed dairy products, which resulted in fermentative enteritis (left prefemoral approach, CO_2 insufflation). (*B*) Retained, inspissated yolk sac (y) in a juvenile radiated tortoise that presented for intermittent anorexia and poor growth. Clinicopathology and diagnostic imaging were unremarkable but endoscope-assisted removal proved curative (left prefemoral approach, CO_2 insufflation). (*C*) Chronic hepatic fibrosis in a green iguana that presented for anorexia and occasional regurgitation. Diagnostic imaging was unremarkable, and the only clinicopathologic abnormality was mild elevation of postprandial bile acids. Endoscopic biopsy confirmed the diagnosis of severe hepatic fibrosis with cholestasis (left lateral coelioscopy, CO_2 insufflation). (*D*) Pale liver (l) in an aldabra tortoise that presented with intermittent anorexia. All liver parameters were unremarkable, but severe hepatic lipidosis was diagnosed after liver biopsy (left prefemoral approach, CO_2 insufflation). (*E*) Diffuse hepatomegaly (l) in a green iguana that presented with lethargy and anorexia. Diagnostic imaging and liver biochemistry were unremarkable; however, moderate leukocytosis, predominantly heterophilia and azurophilia, was evident. Endoscopic liver biopsy confirmed the diagnosis as bacterial hepatitis due to *Klebsiella*, and appropriate treatment based on culture and sensitivity results proved curative (left lateral coelioscopy, CO_2 insufflation). (*F*) Biopsy from the edge of the chelonian liver (l) using 1.7-mm biopsy forceps (b) (left prefemoral approach, CO_2 insufflation). (*Courtesy of* Stephen J. Divers, Athens, GA.)

As an example, **Fig. 20** shows effective telescope and cannulae placement sites for performing orchidectomy in iguanids. In general, the telescope is supported by either an assistant or positioning aids, while the surgeon uses the two instruments.

For chelonian endosurgery, all instruments can be operated through a single prefemoral fossa or separate instruments can be triangulated through each fossa. If the target structure is cranial to the bladder and the chelonian is less than 25–50 kg, it is often preferable for one instrument and telescope to be inserted through one prefemoral fossa, while the second instrument is inserted through the contralateral fossa. For these procedures, the animal is in dorsal recumbency, and instruments are widely

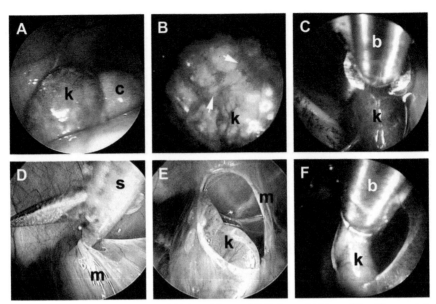

Fig. 19. Endoscopic pathology and kidney biopsy. (*A*) Enlarged kidney (k) with associated renal cyst (c) in a green iguana that presented with anorexia and cachexia. Radiography and ultrasonography confirmed renomegaly, whereas plasma biochemistry showed reversed calcium:phosphorus ratio and elevated uric acid. Endoscopic biopsy confirmed the diagnosis of glomerulonephrosis with renal gout and mineralization (left lateral coelioscopy, CO_2 insufflation). (*B*) Abnormal kidney (k) with fibrous bands (*arrows*) in a female Greek tortoise that presented with anorexia, lethargy, and polyuria. Diagnostic imaging and clinicopathology were unremarkable; however, renal biopsy confirmed the diagnosis as severe tubulonephrosis (left prefemoral approach, CO_2 insufflation). (*C*) Biopsy of an iguanid kidney (k) using 1.7-mm biopsy forceps (b) (right lateral coelioscopy, CO_2 insufflation). (*D*) Incising the caudodorsal coelomic membrane (m) of a yellow-bellied slider using 1.7-mm endoscopy scissors (s) to gain access to the retrocoelomic kidney (left prefemoral approach, CO_2 insufflation). (*E*) View of the incised coelomic membrane (m) showing the kidney (k) (left prefemoral approach, CO_2 insufflation). (*F*) Biopsy forceps (b) being passed through the incision to collect a biopsy from the kidney (k) (left prefemoral approach, CO_2 insufflation). (*Courtesy of* Stephen J. Divers, Athens, GA.)

separated and can be more easily triangulated in front of the bladder. However, for larger chelonians, it can be difficult to impossible for a single surgeon to operate both instruments, while visualization and manipulation of caudal structures (eg, kidney, gonad, adrenal, cloaca) can be severely hampered by the bladder, thereby necessitating a single fossa approach. In large chelonians and those in which a caudal structure is the focus of the procedure, entry through a single prefemoral fossa may be preferable. In these cases, the chelonian may be positioned in dorsal or lateral recumbency, which often provides greater accessibility because the intestines and bladder fall to the dependent areas of the coelom. The telescope and instruments are inserted through the same prefemoral fossa (**Fig. 21**). This approach is easier in animals with a large prefemoral fossa, although the close placement and parallel nature of the instruments still makes triangulation more difficult. In addition, making a single large prefemoral incision for the insertion of all devices is often easier, rather than placing three cannulae adjacent to one another.

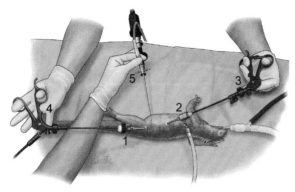

Fig. 20. Diagram showing the positioning for orchidectomy in the iguana. The cannulae are placed caudad, just cranial to the pelvic limb (1) and craniad through an intercostal space (2). The right-handed surgeon uses forceps in the left hand (3) and monopolar scissors in the right (4). An assistant supports the telescope and camera (5). (*Courtesy of* Stephen J. Divers, Athens, GA.)

Iguanid Orchidectomy

With the iguana in right lateral recumbency, the telescope and protection sheath are inserted through the umbilical scar in the ventral midline, just caudal to the anastomosis of the left and right pelvic veins as they form the ventral abdominal vein. The first cannula is placed through the third to last intercostal space, just ventral to the epaxial muscles. The second trocar is placed through the caudodorsal paralumbar fossa, just cranial to the pelvic limb (**Fig. 22**). Grasping forceps are inserted through the cranial port and used to elevate the testis, while scissors (attached to monopolar radiosurgery) are inserted through the caudal port and used to coagulate and cut through

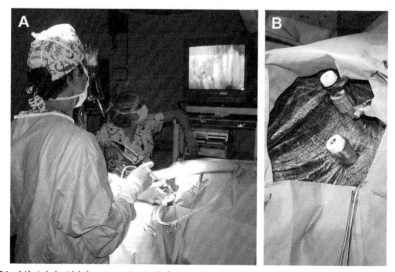

Fig. 21. (*A*) Adult Aldabra tortoise in left lateral recumbency having right prefemoral endosurgery performed. (*B*) Close-up view of the surgical site showing the placement of two 6-mm Ternamian endotip cannulae. (*Courtesy of* Stephen J. Divers, Athens, GA.)

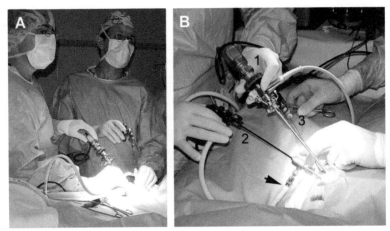

Fig. 22. (*A*) Endoscopic orchidectomy performed in a green iguana. (*B*) Close-up of the surgical site showing the placement of the telescope (1), 3-mm forceps (2), and 3-mm bipolar forceps (3). Note that the insufflation line is connected to one of the cannulae (*arrow*). (*Courtesy of* Stephen J. Divers, Athens, GA.)

the mesorchium and associated vessels (**Fig. 23**A–C). In larger iguanas, bipolar forceps are used to coagulate blood vessels before sharp dissection. The testis is extracted through the caudal cannula incision, which can be enlarged if necessary (**Fig. 23**D). The cannula holes are closed with a single suture or tissue adhesive. The iguana is rotated into left lateral recumbency, and using the same telescope entry site, the procedure is repeated for the second testis.

Chelonian Ovariectomy/Oophorectomy

Because endoscope-assisted oophorectomy is covered elsewhere in this issue, this article focuses on true endosurgical oophorectomy. To date this has been performed on 50- to 80-kg hybrid Galapagos tortoises using 5-mm instrumentation, but no fundamental reason exists why the same technique could not be used with 3-mm instruments in smaller animals. The immature ovary is positioned close to the kidney in the caudodorsal coelom, making visualizing both ovaries from a single prefemoral approach impossible because of the bladder. With the animal in lateral recumbency, a large prefemoral approach to the coelom is made to accommodate the telescope and two instruments through a single incision; cannulae are generally not helpful because the instruments are so closely aligned (**Fig. 24**A). The ovary is identified and elevated away from the serosal surface using Babcock or Kelly forceps, and monopolar scissors are used to dissect the ovary free from its mesovarian attachments (**Fig. 24**B). The prefemoral incision is closed routinely and the procedure repeated on the opposite side.

COMPLICATIONS

The major complications encountered are typically associated with anesthesia and the advanced disease state of many presented reptiles. The importance of a thorough preoperative evaluation and stabilization cannot be overemphasized. Ventilation, fluid support, and temperature maintenance are critical. Minor hemorrhage after tissue biopsy is common but clinically insignificant. Most endoscopy issues are related to

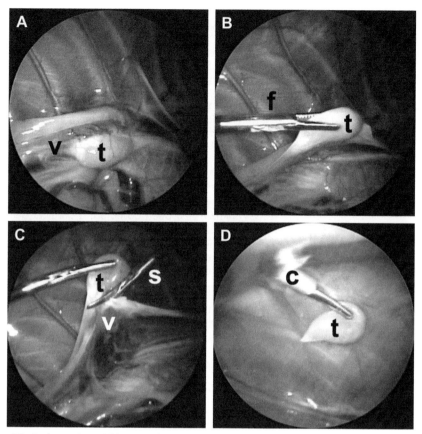

Fig. 23. Endoscopic orchidectomy in a green iguana (right lateral coelioscopy). (*A*) Endoscopic view of the mid-dorsal coelom, right testis (t) and closely associated renal vein (v). (*B*) The testis (t) is grasped and elevated away from the body wall and associated structures using 3-mm forceps (f). (*C*) The mesorchium and associated vessels are carefully coagulated and incised between the testis (t) and renal vein (v) using monopolar scissors (s), taking care to avoid the adrenal gland. (*D*) The 3.5-mm cannula (c) is slid up the shaft of the forceps enabling the testis (t) to be removed through the skin and muscle incision (not through the cannula). (*Courtesy of* Stephen J. Divers, Athens, GA.)

operator error until experience and ability have been gained. In general, the ability to examine reptiles internally and collect tissue samples greatly aids diagnosis and improves treatment success. To facilitate endoscopy caseload without compromising patient welfare, surgeons are recommended to obtain training and retain the option of converting to a traditional surgical approach if required.

POSTOPERATIVE CARE

Reptiles should be closely supervised until ambulatory, and be continuously maintained within their species-specific preferred optimum temperature zone. Meloxicam is relied on postoperatively, although opiates and local anesthetics could prove useful as part of a balanced approach to analgesia. Continued fluid therapy is more important than an immediate return to feeding. Typically, reptiles return to normal function

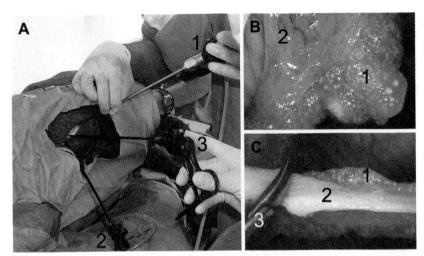

Fig. 24. Endoscopic oophorectomy in an immature female Galapagos tortoise. (*A*) Close-up of the surgical site showing the single prefemoral incision that accommodates the telescope (1) that is held by an assistant, while the surgeon uses the monopolar scissors (2) and grasping forceps (3). (*B*) Endoscopic view of the immature ovary (1) and vascular mesovarium (2). (*C*) Endoscopic view of the ovary (1) being elevated away from the body wall thereby stretching the mesovarium (2) and facilitating coagulation and incision by monopolar scissors (3). (*Courtesy of* Stephen J. Divers, Athens, GA.)

and behaviors quicker after endoscopic procedures than traditional surgeries. Sutures are removed at 6 to 8 weeks.

OUTCOME

Return to normal behaviors and weight gain are often the most useful indicators of improvement. Serial clinicopathology can also be useful if abnormalities were detected preoperatively. Serial endoscopic evaluations can be used to monitor patients, especially because some diseases (eg, hepatic lipidosis, glomerulonephrosis) may have a protracted course.

REFERENCES

1. Ackermann J, Carpenter JW. Using endoscopy to remove a gastric foreign body in a python. Vet Med 1995;90:761–3.
2. Burrows CF, Heard DJ. Endoscopy in nondomestic species. In: Tams TR, editor. Small animal endoscopy. St. Louis (MO): Mosby; 1999. p. 297–321.
3. Cooper JE. Endoscopy in exotic species. In: Brearley MJ, Cooper JE, Sullivan M, editors. Color atlas of small animal endoscopy. St. Louis (MO): Mosby; 1991. p. 111–22.
4. Coppoolse KJ, Zwart P. Cloacoscopy in reptiles. Vet Q 1985;7(3):243–5.
5. Pressler BM, Goodman RA, Harms CA, et al. Endoscopic evaluation of the esophagus and stomach in three loggerhead sea turtles (*Caretta caretta*) and a Malaysian giant turtle (*Orlitia borneensis*). J Zoo Wildl Med 2003;34(1):88–92.
6. Lafortune M, Göbel T, Jacobson E, et al. Respiratory bronchoscopy of subadult american alligators (*Alligator mississippiensis*) and tracheal wash evaluation. J Zoo Wildl Med 2005;36(1):12–20.

7. Hernandez-Divers SJ, Stahl S, Hernandez-Divers SM, et al. Coelomic endoscopy of the green iguana (*Iguana iguana*). J Herp Med Surg 2004;14:10–8.

8. Hernandez-Divers SJ, Stahl S, Stedman NL, et al. Renal evaluation in the green iguana (*Iguana iguana*): assessment of plasma biochemistry, glomerular filtration rate, and endoscopic biopsy. J Zoo Wildl Med 2005;36:155–68.

9. Hernandez-Divers SJ, Stahl SJ, Farrell R. Endoscopic gender identification of hatchling Chinese box turtles (*Cuora flavomarginata*) under local and general anesthesia. J Am Vet Med Assoc 2009;234(6):800–4.

10. Hernandez-Divers SJ, Stahl SJ, McBride M, et al. Evaluation of an endoscopic liver biopsy technique in green iguanas. J Am Vet Med Assoc 2007;230(12): 1849–53.

11. Stahl SJ, Hernandez-Divers SJ, Cooper TL, et al. Evaluation of transcutaneous pulmonoscopy for examination and biopsy of the lungs of ball pythons and determination of preferred biopsy specimen handling and fixation procedures. J Am Vet Med Assoc 2008;233(3):440–5.

12. Hernandez-Divers SJ. Diagnostic and surgical endoscopy. In: Raiti P, Girling S, editors. Manual of reptiles. Cheltenham (England): British Small Animal Veterinary Association; 2004. p. 103–14.

13. Hernandez-Divers SJ, Hernandez-Divers SM, Wilson GH, et al. A review of reptile diagnostic coelioscopy. J Herp Med Surg 2005;15:16–31.

14. Innis C, Hernandez-Divers SJ, Martinez-Jimenez D. Coelioscopic-assisted prefemoral oophorectomy in chelonians. J Am Vet Med Assoc 2007;230:1049–52.

15. Hernandez-Divers SJ. Endoscopic renal evaluation and biopsy of Chelonia. Vet Rec 2004;154(3):73–80.

16. Hernandez-Divers SJ. Minimally-invasive endoscopic surgery of birds. J Avian Med Surg 2005;19(2):107–20.

17. Mader DR. Reptile medicine and surgery. 2nd edition. St Louis (MO): Elsevier; 2006.

18. Raiti P, Girling S. Manual of reptiles. 2nd edition. Cheltenham (England): British Small Animal Veterinary Association; 2004.

19. Martinez-Jimenez D, Hernandez-Divers SJ. Emergency care of reptiles. Vet Clin North Am Exot Anim Pract 2007;10(2):557–85.

20. Schumacher J, Yelen T. Anesthesia and analgesia. In: Mader DR, editor. Reptile medicine and surgery. St Louis (MO): Elsevier; 2006. p. 442–52.

21. Rostal D, Grumbles J, Lance V, et al. Non-lethal sexing techniques for hatchling and immature desert tortoises (*Gopherus agassizii*). Herp Mono 1994;8: 103–16.

22. Sladky KK, Kinney ME, Johnson SM. Analgesic efficacy of butorphanol and morphine in bearded dragons and corn snakes. J Am Vet Med Assoc 2008; 233(2):267–73.

23. Sladky KK, Miletic V, Paul-Murphy J, et al. Analgesic efficacy and respiratory effects of butorphanol and morphine in turtles. J Am Vet Med Assoc 2007;230: 1356–62.

24. Hernandez-Divers SJ, Papich M, McBride M, et al. Intravenous and oral pharmacokinetics of meloxicam in the green iguana (*Iguana iguana*). Am J Vet Res 2009, in press.

25. Hernandez-Divers SJ, Shearer D. Pulmonary mycobacteriosis caused by *Mycobacterium haemophilum* and *M. marinum* in a royal python. J Am Vet Med Assoc 2002;220(11):1661–3.

26. Taylor WM. Endoscopy. In: Mader DR, editor. Reptile medicine and surgery. St. Louis (MO): Elsevier; 2006. p. 549–63.

27. Jekl V, Knotek Z. Endoscopic examination of snakes by access through an air sac. Vet Rec 2006;158(12):407.
28. Tams TR. Small animal endoscopy. 2nd edition. St Louis (MO): Mosby; 1999. 497.
29. McCarthy TC. Veterinary endoscopy for the small animal practitioner. St Louis (MO): Elsevier; 2005. 624.
30. Monnet E, Twedt DC. Laparoscopy. Vet Clin North Am Small Anim Pract 2003; 33(5):1147–63.
31. Lhermette P, Sobel D. Bsava manual of canine and feline endoscopy and endo-surgery. 1st edition. Cheltenham (England): British Small Animal Veterinary Association; 2008. 234.
32. Falcone RE, Wanamaker SR, Barnes F, et al. Laparoscopic vs. open wedge biopsy of the liver. J Laparoendosc Surg 1993;3(4):325–9.
33. Golditch IM. Laparoscopy: advances and advantages. Fertil Steril 1971;22(5): 306–10.
34. Grauer GF, Twedt DC, Mero KN. Evaluation of laparoscopy for obtaining renal biopsy specimens from dogs and cats. J Am Vet Med Assoc 1983;183(6):677–9.
35. Hancock RB, Lanz OI, Waldron DR, et al. Comparison of postoperative pain after ovariohysterectomy by harmonic scalpel-assisted laparoscopy compared with median celiotomy and ligation in dogs. Vet Surg 2005;34:273–82.
36. Kehlet H. Surgical stress response: does endoscopic surgery confer an advantage? World J Surg 1999;23(8):801–7.
37. Lagares-Garcia JA, Bansidhar B, Moore RA. Benefits of laparoscopy in middle-aged patients. Surg Endosc 2003;17(1):68–72.
38. Orlando R, Lirussi F, Okolicsanyi L. Laparoscopy and liver biopsy: further evidence that the two procedures improve the diagnosis of liver cirrhosis. A retrospective study of 1,003 consecutive examinations. J Clin Gastroenterol 1990; 12(1):47–52.
39. Rawlings CA, Diamond H, Howerth EW, et al. Diagnostic quality of percutaneous kidney biopsy specimens obtained with laparoscopy versus ultrasound guidance in dogs. J Am Vet Med Assoc 2003;223(3):317–21.
40. Reissman P, Gofrit O, Rivkind A. Exploratory laparoscopy: a crucial advantage of laparoscopic over standard appendectomy. South Med J 1994;87(5):576.
41. Vander Velpen GC, Shimi SM, Cuschieri A. Diagnostic yield and management benefit of laparoscopy: a prospective audit. Gut 1994;35(11):1617–21.
42. Weickert U, Buttmann A, Jakobs R, et al. Diagnosis of liver cirrhosis: a comparison of modified ultrasound and laparoscopy in 100 consecutive patients. J Clin Gastroenterol 2005;39(6):529–32.
43. Yu SY, Chiu JH, Loong CC, et al. Diagnostic laparoscopy: indication and benefit. Zhonghua Yi Xue Za Zhi (Taipei) 1997;59(3):158–63.
44. Hernandez-Divers SJ. Surgery: principles and techniques. In: Raiti P, Girling S, editors. Manual of reptiles. Cheltenham (England): British Small Animal Veterinary Association; 2004. p. 147–67.
45. Divers SJ. Lizard endoscopic techniques with particular regard to the green iguana (*Iguana iguana*). Semin Avian Exotic Pet Med 1999;8:122–9.
46. Hernandez-Divers SJ, Innis C. Renal disease in reptiles: diagnosis and clinical management. In: Mader DR, editor. Reptile medicine and surgery. St Louis (MO): Elsevier; 2006. p. 878–92.

Endoscopy and Endosurgery of the Chelonian Reproductive Tract

Charles J. Innis, VMD

KEYWORDS

- Turtle • Tortoise • Chelonian • Endoscopy
- Surgery • Reproductive

Captive breeding of chelonians has become more common in recent years because of increased popularity of reptiles as pets, as well as the need for captive breeding for conservation purposes. In addition, numerous in situ turtle conservation projects have been developed to improve the reproductive success of wild populations. In many locations, wild gravid female turtles are injured by automobiles during nesting excursions. As a result of these developments, veterinarians are increasingly involved in chelonian gender identification studies, management of female reproductive disorders, and infertility investigations.

Endosurgery and endoscopic-assisted surgery are being used with increasing frequency in veterinary medicine, including zoologic medicine.[1–4] Such techniques provide excellent visualization, are minimally invasive, reduce surgical trauma, and result in faster healing and recovery.[5,6] In reptiles, endoscopy has been used diagnostically for more than 20 years, although more detailed descriptions and objective evaluations have only recently been conducted.[3,4] Endoscopic surgery involves the use of a telescopic lens system and endosurgical instruments to evaluate and manipulate tissues, and perform surgery within the body cavity of the patient. Endoscopic-assisted surgery involves the use of endoscopic visualization and endosurgical instruments to evaluate, manipulate, and exteriorize tissue, with the definitive surgery performed outside of the body cavity. For chelonians, endoscopy of the coelom (coelioscopy) and the cloaca (cloacoscopy) allows access to the reproductive tract, and has reduced the need for more invasive surgical approaches such as plastron osteotomy.[4,7,8]

Several reviews of chelonian reproductive disorders have been published.[7,9–11] Reproductive disorders such as oophoritis, salpingitis, follicular stasis, retained eggs, dystocia, ectopic eggs, and oviduct prolapse are common in female

Animal Health Department, New England Aquarium, Central Wharf, Boston, MA 02110, USA
E-mail address: cinnis@neaq.org

Vet Clin Exot Anim 13 (2010) 243–254
doi:10.1016/j.cvex.2010.01.005
1094-9194/10/$ – see front matter © 2010 Elsevier Inc. All rights reserved.

chelonians.[4,7,9–15] The techniques described in this article assume familiarity with such disorders, and assume that the clinician has formulated a proper diagnostic and treatment plan. The clinician should use common sense and standard medical judgment to determine the course of action, and must be familiar with normal clutch sizes and egg sizes for various species. If true obstructive dystocia, oviduct adhesions, abnormally large eggs, or ectopic eggs are present, induction of oviposition is not indicated and surgical management is needed. For example, if a female has obvious structural abnormalities of the pelvis that will not allow for normal oviposition, use of drugs to promote oviduct contraction is contraindicated. In such cases, oophorectomy should be considered in addition to surgical management of the immediate dystocia. Eggs have been found in the coelom, urinary bladder, and colon of turtles, in which case medical induction of oviposition will not be helpful.[8,9,14,15]

GENERAL CHELONIAN ANATOMY AND REPRODUCTION

Chelonians have paired gonads located in the dorsal caudal coelom anterior to the kidneys. Females have paired ovaries and oviducts. Mature, yolk-filled ovarian follicles develop periodically (often seasonally). After ovulation, ova enter the oviduct where they are fertilized, and the albumen, shell membranes, and eggshell are produced. The oviducts exit into the dorsal lateral cloaca. Males have paired testes and a single phallus. The phallus is located within the cloaca and serves only as a conduit for semen, having no urinary function.

Shelled eggs are held in the oviducts before oviposition. In some sea turtles, eggs may be in the oviduct for as little as 9 days,[16] whereas the chicken turtle (*Deirochelys reticularia*) normally retains eggs in the oviducts for 4 to 6 months.[17] On average, however, most species retain eggs for 1 to 2 months before oviposition. Prolonged egg retention in captivity may indicate some pathologic condition, lack of suitable nesting sites, or other stressor.

Clutch size, egg size, egg type, and nesting frequency vary among species. Pancake tortoises (*Malacochersus tornieri*), bowsprit tortoises (*Chersina angulata*), spider tortoises (*Pyxis arachnoides*), black-breasted leaf turtles (*Geomyda spengleri*), Sulawesi forest turtles (*Leucocephalon yuwonoi*), and Central American wood turtles (*Rhinoclemmys* spp) generally produce only 1 (rarely 2) very large egg(s) per clutch, but may nest several times per year. At the other extreme, the large sea turtles, snapping turtles (*Chelydra serpentina* and *Macroclemys temmincki*), and softshell turtles (*Trionyx* sp, *Apalone* sp, and others) may lay dozens of eggs per clutch, with some of the sea turtles nesting several times per year. Eggs have either calcareous hard shells, or flexible leathery shells depending on the species.

EQUIPMENT

Rigid endoscopes in the range of 1.9 to 10 mm in diameter are used for chelonian coelioscopy and cloacoscopy, depending on the size of the patient. Flexible scopes may also be of use for cloacoscopy. Although scopes can be operated by looking directly into the eye piece, the use of an endocamera and video monitor system is preferred to allow for better posture, video documentation, and teaching. The smaller telescope systems are generally equipped with a sheath to protect the scope and to allow introduction of biopsy forceps, endoscopic surgical instruments, irrigation, and insufflation. Larger scopes may be introduced via cannulae. In some cases, 2 or 3 cannulae may be placed into the coelom to allow for endosurgical techniques using multiple instruments under endoscopic visualization. Various types of endoscopic biopsy instruments, scissors, sealers, dividers, grasping forceps, ligation clips, and aspiration needles may be used depending on the skill of the operator and clinical situation.

For good visualization, insufflation of the coelom may be needed to allow adequate spatial separation of organs. If available, the ideal insufflator is a purpose built carbon dioxide endosurgical insufflator. Carbon dioxide is less likely to cause gas emboli than air. In addition, the intracoelomic pressure is precisely regulated by the insufflator, which replaces gas when the pressure falls, and stops gas flow when the desired pressure is achieved. In most cases, intracoelomic pressures of 3 to 5 mm Hg are safe for chelonians. If an endosurgical insufflator is not available, a simple aquarium air pump may be used to insufflate the coelom. In some cases, the surgeon may choose to use sterile saline for insufflation. In both cases, the flow of air or saline must be carefully regulated to prevent over-inflation leading to cardiorespiratory depression. The flow of air or saline may be adjusted using the sheath or cannula ports to which the pump or fluid line is attached. Postoperatively, gas should be evacuated from the coelom to reduce the potential of buoyancy disorders, air embolism, and postoperative discomfort.

To sterilize endoscopes, cold sterilization products or gas sterilization may be used. Some modern telescopes may be autoclaved, but manufacturers' instructions should be followed closely. Similarly, because most endoscopes and endoscopic instruments are very expensive and delicate, all manufacturers' handling, cleaning, disinfection, sterilization, and storage instructions should be followed carefully.

GENERAL APPROACH FOR CHELONIAN COELIOSCOPY

Surgical access to the reproductive tract of chelonia has traditionally been achieved via plastron osteotomy and the creation of a bone flap.[18] Although this technique has been used successfully for many years, it is more invasive than soft tissue approaches. In addition, healing can be prolonged (months to years) and in some cases sequestration of the replaced osteotomy bone flap may occur (Innis, personal observation, 2004). As an alternative to plastron osteotomy, soft tissue coeliotomy is less invasive, with rapid skin and muscle healing.[4,19] Prefemoral coeliotomy has been used for intestinal, urinary bladder, and reproductive tract surgery in chelonia.[4,13,20,21] Access to the anterior coelom of sea turtles has also been achieved via an axillary or supraplastron approach, although to the author's knowledge these anterior approaches have not yet been reported in freshwater turtles or tortoises.[19,22] It is likely that soft tissue approaches to the coelom are less painful than plastron osteotomy, although controlled studies are lacking.

For chelonian surgery, adequate supportive care, analgesia, and anesthesia must be provided, with appropriate monitoring of cardiorespiratory function. Although some investigators have reported using only local anesthesia for chelonian coelioscopy, this likely provides inadequate analgesia for more involved coelioscopic procedures.[23] In a recent comparison of local versus general anesthesia for chelonian coelioscopy, objective anesthetic scores were significantly better for procedures conducted with general anesthesia.[24]

For coelioscopy, the turtle is positioned with consideration of normal chelonian anatomy and the goals of the procedure. For best visualization of more dorsal organs such as the lung, gonad, or kidney, positioning the patient in lateral or oblique recumbency may be useful. However, several successful laparoscopic-assisted procedures of chelonia have been performed with the patient in dorsal recumbency, as discussed later. The hind limb of the turtle is positioned in extension to expose the prefemoral fossa (**Fig. 1**). The prefemoral region and surrounding shell is aseptically prepared

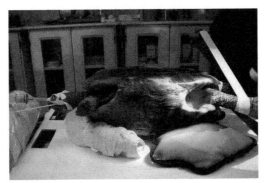

Fig. 1. Prefemoral surgical approach to the chelonian coelom. The hind leg is restrained in extension. (*Courtesy of* Charles J. Innis, VMD, Boston, MA.)

and surgically draped, and a craniocaudal skin incision is made in the center of the prefemoral fossa (**Fig. 2**A). An inappropriately located incision may result in exposure of the anterior femur, posterior surface of the kidney, lung, or pelvis, or may simply result in tunneling along the carapace or plastron. To avoid this, the surgeon should be familiar with chelonian anatomy, and should palpate the surrounding structures (eg, flex and extend the hind limb) before making the incision. The size of the incision is dependent on the goal of the procedure (ie, examination only vs surgical manipulation). Longer incisions often provide better visualization of the coelomic aponeurosis, resulting in faster access to the coelom, and less frustration for the surgeon. The

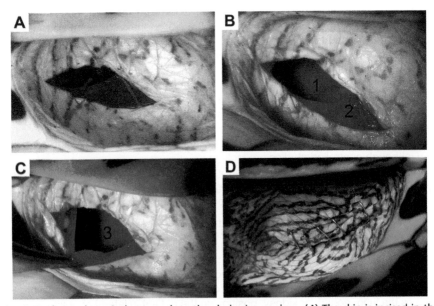

Fig. 2. Prefemoral surgical approach to the chelonian coelom. (*A*) The skin is incised in the center of the prefemoral space. (*B*) The aponeurosis (1) of the transverse and oblique abdominal muscles (2) is exposed. (*C*) The aponeurosis and coelomic peritoneum are incised to enter the coelom. Note the surface of the liver (3). (*D*) Prefemoral skin incision closed with skin staples. (*Courtesy of* Charles J. Innis, VMD, Boston, MA.)

subcutaneous connective tissue and fat are dissected to expose the tendinous aponeurosis of the transverse and oblique abdominal muscles (**Fig. 2**B), and the aponeurosis and coelomic membrane are incised to enter the coelom (**Fig. 2**C). Some surgeons prefer to use blunt dissection for much of the prefemoral approach, including blunt penetration of the aponeurosis and coelomic membrane,[24] but the author prefers a combination of blunt and sharp dissection, with incision of the aponeurosis and membrane made sharply under direct visualization with the aponeurosis held with forceps. In the author's experience, blunt methods may fail to penetrate the coelomic membrane, resulting in an obscured endoscopic examination (**Fig. 3**A). If properly performed, incision of the membrane and introduction of the endoscope into the coelom should result in a perfectly clear view of the viscera, leaving no question whether the surgeon has actually entered the coelom (**Fig. 3**B).

On completion of surgery, closure of the coelomic aponeurosis and peritoneum is performed using absorbable suture in a simple interrupted or continuous pattern. Skin closure may be performed using suture or skin staples (see **Fig. 2**D). In very small turtles with very small incisions (eg, hatchlings for gender identification), incisions may be closed with surgical tissue glue; however, tissue adhesive may not always maintain good closure and cases of dehiscence have been seen.[24] When skin sutures or staples are used, full access to water may be provided for aquatic turtles 24 hours after prefemoral coeliotomy.[4] If tissue adhesive is used, turtles are not provided full access to water for 48 hours. Skin healing is often complete within 4 to 8 weeks.[4]

COELIOSCOPIC GENDER IDENTIFICATION

Sexual dimorphism is usually apparent in adult chelonians. General guidelines for identification of males include a longer tail with a more distal cloacal opening than females, and a plastral concavity to facilitate mating. These rules do not hold true for all species and other species-specific traits may be noted. For example, sexual dimorphisms may be seen in the eye or skin color, adult size, or toenail length of

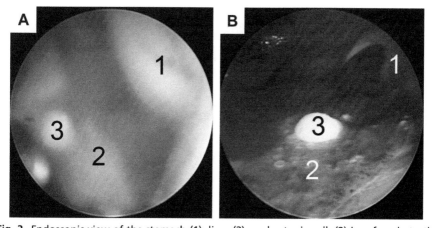

Fig. 3. Endoscopic view of the stomach (1), liver (2), and ectopic yolk (3) in a female turtle using a right prefemoral approach with the patient in dorsal recumbency. (*A*) Obscured view as seen through the translucent coelomic peritoneum. The endoscope has not entered the coelom. (*B*) Clear view obtained after proper entry into the coelom. The stomach, liver, and ectopic yolk are clearly visible. Note the pathologic craterlike lesions on the surface of the liver. (*Courtesy of* Charles J. Innis, VMD, Boston, MA.)

some species. In hatchling or juvenile turtles, however, there are generally no external features that allow for gender identification. Coelioscopic examination of the gonad may provide accurate gender identification in such animals.[23,24] Immature follicles are visible on the ovary of immature females of most chelonian species (**Fig. 4**A); the testicle tends to be smoother and more vascular (**Fig. 4**B). Although not yet validated in comparison with gonad examination, cloacoscopy could prove useful for visualization of the phallus in the cloaca of juvenile male turtles. However, a clitoris-like structure resembling the phallus may be seen in the cloaca of some adult female tortoises. Thus, future blinded studies should compare and validate gender identification obtained via gonad examination versus cloacoscopy in juvenile chelonians.

COELIOSCOPIC-ASSISTED SURGERY

Eleven cases of coelioscopic-assisted reproductive surgery of chelonia (management of retained eggs, ectopic eggs, oviduct prolapse, or elective oophorectomy) were recently reported, with an average surgical time of 30 to 40 minutes.[4] Species included a Gulf Coast box turtle (*Terrapene carolina major*), red-eared slider (*Trachemys scripta elegans*), eastern painted turtle (*Chrysemys picta picta*), four-eyed turtle (*Sacalia bealei*), and Chinese red-necked pond turtle (*Chinemys kwantungensis*).

For oophorectomy, salpingectomy, or salpingotomy, turtles are placed in dorsal recumbency, and prefemoral coeliotomy is performed. The endoscope is introduced into the coelom and the reproductive tract is identified. Endoscopic grasping forceps are passed alongside the endoscope into the coelom to facilitate manipulation of the reproductive tract. For oophorectomy an avascular area of ovarian interfollicular connective tissue is selected for placement of the grasping forceps, taking care to avoid rupture of ovarian follicles (**Fig. 5**A). Gentle traction is applied under endoscopic visualization, and the ovary is cautiously retracted toward the coelomic incision. With the ovary held just deep to the prefemoral incision, the endoscope is removed and the

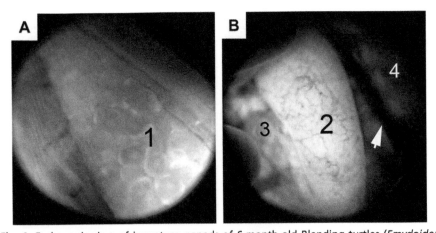

Fig. 4. Endoscopic view of immature gonads of 6-month-old Blanding turtles (*Emydoidea blandingii*). (*A*) Spherical immature follicles are clearly visible on the ovary (1). (*Courtesy of* Eric Baitchman, DVM, Boston, MA.) (*B*) The surface of the testicle (2) is relatively smooth and more vascular than the ovary. The adrenal gland (3), kidney (4), and large renal vein (*arrow*) are also visible in close proximity to the gonad. (*Courtesy of* Charles J. Innis, VMD, Boston, MA.)

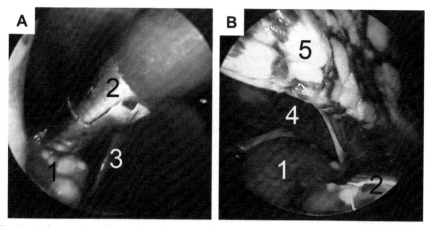

Fig. 5. Prefemoral coelioscopic-assisted oophorectomy of a mature turtle with patient in dorsal recumbency. (*A*) Right prefemoral endoscopic view of the ovary (1) being retracted with endoscopic grasping forceps (2). A margin of the liver (3) is visible anterior to the ovary. (*B*) Exteriorization of the ovary. Grasping forceps (2) are used to carefully withdraw ovarian follicles (1) through the incised aponeurosis (4). The ventral border of the skin incision is visible (5). (*Courtesy of* Charles J. Innis, VMD, Boston, MA.)

ovarian follicles are gently exteriorized (**Fig. 5**B). In some cases, numerous large ovarian follicles are present, and the coelomic incision may need to be extended. Rarely, fine-needle aspiration of individual follicles may be required to reduce follicle size. Exteriorization is continued until all follicles are visible and clear cranial and caudal borders of the mesovarium are visible (**Fig. 6**A). The ovarian vasculature is ligated with stainless steel surgical ligation clips or suture, and the mesovarium is transected (**Fig. 6**B). Coelioscopic examination of the ligation sites is performed to verify hemostasis and to verify complete excision of all ovarian tissue. In cases in which bilateral oophorectomy is desired, the second ovary can often be exteriorized and resected via the same prefemoral incision as the first. Thus, bilateral

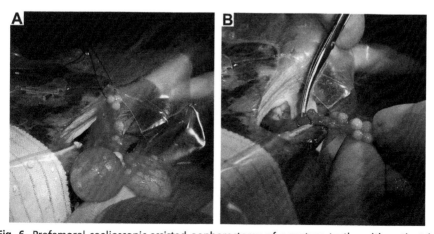

Fig. 6. Prefemoral coelioscopic-assisted oophorectomy of a mature turtle, with patient in dorsal recumbency. (*A*) The ovary has been completely exteriorized. (*B*) The mesovarium and associated vasculature is ligated and transected. (*Courtesy of* Charles J. Innis, VMD, Boston, MA.)

oophorectomy may be achieved via a unilateral incision. If needed, a contralateral incision can be made for additional access.

Given the common risk of reproductive tract disease and the relative simplicity of coelioscopic-assisted oophorectomy, the author recommends prophylactic coelio-scopic-assisted oophorectomy as a practical and safe option for sterilizing mature female chelonians. Selection of turtles for coelioscopic-assisted oophorectomy should be limited to mature females, because the ovaries of immature females are more closely adhered to the dorsal coelom, and the mesovarium may not have enough laxity to allow exteriorization. In these patients, a true coelioscopic oophorectomy (using endosurgical hemostasis and excision) would be required. The author has not yet had occasion to attempt coelioscopic-assisted oophorectomy in any species of tortoise, and it is possible that the anatomic differences among species may limit the applicability of this method in all situations.

Coelioscopic surgery or coelioscopic-assisted surgery may also be used for removal of ectopic eggs from the coelom, salpingotomy for removal of eggs from the oviduct, or salpingectomy for removal of diseased or necrotic oviducts.[4] The principles are identical to those used for oophorectomy, including coelioscopic visualization, manipulation, exteriorization, and vascular ligation (**Figs. 7** and **8**). In some cases, eggs may need to be fractured or aspirated for removal if they are larger than the available prefemoral space. Some female chelonians have a hinged plastron or some flexibility of the caudal plastron, and retractors may be used to increase the available prefemoral space. Whether or not to fracture or aspirate an egg is at the discretion of the surgeon, and will partly depend on the egg type (hard-shelled or leathery), number of eggs, and risk of coelomic contamination. Thorough isolation of the oviduct (similar to isolation of bowel for enterotomy), suction, and lavage may facilitate safe removal of eggs. Hemi-oophor-osalpingectomy may be considered for cases of unilateral ovarian or oviduct pathology, with the goal of maintaining future reproductive potential.[13]

It is likely that additional coelioscopic reproductive surgical procedures (eg, true endosurgical oophorectomy, vasectomy, or castration) will be perfected for chelonia in the near future as the skills of veterinary endosurgeons continue to improve.

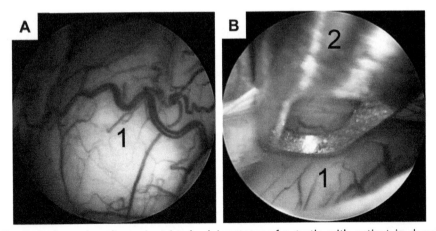

Fig. 7. Prefemoral coelioscopic-assisted salpingotomy of a turtle with patient in dorsal recumbency. (*A*) Endoscopic view of an egg (*1*) retained within the oviduct. (*B*) The oviduct adjacent to the egg (1) is grasped with endoscopic forceps (2). (*Courtesy of* Charles J. Innis, VMD, Boston, MA.)

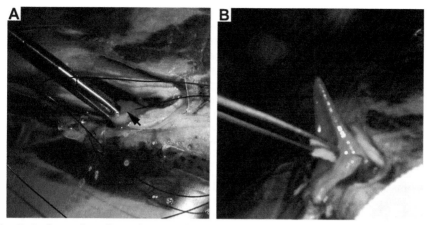

Fig. 8. Prefemoral coelioscopic-assisted salpingotomy of a turtle with patient in dorsal recumbency. (*A*) The oviduct (*arrow*) is exteriorized and held in place with stay sutures. (*B*) Salpingotomy and fragmentation of the egg is conducted to remove the egg. (*Courtesy of* Charles J. Innis, VMD, Boston, MA.)

CLOACOSCOPIC TECHNIQUES

Cloacoscopy offers a noninvasive method of evaluation of the reptile reproductive tract. Eggs that are positioned within the pelvic canal or distal oviduct may be visualized and manipulated per cloaca (**Fig. 9**A).[7,8,14,25] A nasal or vaginal speculum attached to a standard otoscope handle may provide visualization of eggs in the distal cloaca. Alternatively, an otoendoscope or small rigid endoscope and operating sheath can be used for excellent visualization of the cloaca. Infusion of saline through the infusion/instrument port of the otoendoscope or endoscope dramatically enhances visualization by distending the cloaca. The oviduct openings are generally located dorsolaterally in the cloaca, adjacent to the urethra and rectum (**Fig. 9**B).

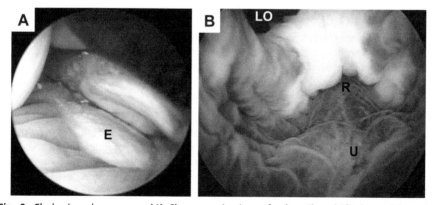

Fig. 9. Chelonian cloacoscopy. (*A*) Cloacoscopic view of a heavily calcified egg (E) at the distal orifice of the oviduct of a tortoise. There is a reflection of the egg as a result of an air-saline interface. The endoscopist's gloved finger is visible to the upper left of the egg, allowing for palpation and manipulation of the egg. (*B*) Cloacoscopy of a female turtle in ventral recumbency using saline infusion. The urethral orifice (U) is visible ventral to the rectal orifice (R). The left oviduct (LO) is visible dorsal and lateral to the rectum. (*Courtesy of* Charles J. Innis, VMD, Boston, MA.)

Cloacoscopic examination may require anesthesia or sedation in some strong specimens, but has been performed without sedation in many cases. Anesthesia should be used, however, if any significant egg manipulation is required. Once the egg is visualized, various techniques can be used to remove it. In general, the cloaca should be lavaged with saline or medical water-soluble lubricant. Soft-shelled eggs may be punctured and aspirated. Hard-shelled eggs may need to be punctured using a drill bit on a rotary tool. Obviously, caution must be used to avoid cloacal or oviduct trauma. Often, once the integrity of a soft-shelled egg is lost, the egg will collapse and be expelled within several minutes, particularly if the female had been recently treated with oxytocin. Hard-shelled eggs may sometimes collapse, but often need to be fragmented for piecemeal removal.

If the egg still does not pass after puncturing, manual extraction of the egg can be attempted. An assistant can provide caudal pressure on the egg by prefemoral palpation, while the veterinarian tries to extract the egg per cloaca under cloacoscopic visualization. Hemostats, alligator forceps, or other grasping instruments may be used, but these instruments often tear the eggshell, and may not allow the egg to be extracted intact. Another option used by the author in several cases is to extract the egg using a Foley urinary catheter. The distal tip of the catheter is cut off, so that the balloon is at the end of the catheter. Before use in the patient, the balloon is filled with air and then emptied to predetermine the amount of air that will be needed to dilate the balloon to the approximate volume of the egg. To provide rigidity to the catheter, the infusion port is filled with water, and the catheter is placed in a freezer for several minutes. Once rigid, the catheter is passed into the cloaca and into the egg. The balloon is filled with air to the predetermined volume, and the air infusion port is clamped with hemostats to prevent escape of the air. Once in position, gentle caudal traction is provided, and the egg is removed intact. Obvious complications such as over inflation and tearing of the oviduct must be considered. The procedure can be repeated over hours to days as needed for subsequent eggs as they move into position, but in some cases, removal of 1 offending egg allows the remainder to pass normally.

Using similar techniques, egg removal from the chelonian bladder has been successfully performed per cloaca.[8] For such cases, saline-infusion cystoscopy is used to identify and isolate the egg, and a variety of techniques (as described earlier) are used to fragment and remove the egg. Thorough lavage of the bladder ensures complete removal of egg fragments and contents. These principles would likely also be effective for eggs found in the colon. It is likely that endoscopic snares or baskets may be useful for retrieving eggs during cloacoscopic visualization.

SUMMARY

The development of endosurgical techniques for chelonians has reduced the need for more invasive techniques. Surgical access and manipulation of much of the coelomic viscera of chelonians can be accomplished using endoscopy. In considering the surgical management of chelonians, the surgeon should strongly consider endoscopic options, and only use plastron osteotomy if absolutely necessary.

ACKNOWLEDGMENTS

The author thanks Drs Clarence Rawlings, Todd Tams, Stephen Divers, Scott Stahl, and the staff of Karl Storz Veterinary Endoscopy for mentorship and technical support in the development of many of the techniques described herein.

REFERENCES

1. Rawlings CA, Foutz TL, Mahaffey MB, et al. A rapid and strong laparoscopic-assisted gastropexy in dogs. Am J Vet Res 2001;62(6):871–5.
2. Hernandez-Divers SJ, Stahl SJ, Wilson GH, et al. Endoscopic orchidectomy and salpingohysterectomy of pigeons (*Columba livia*): an avian model for minimally invasive endosurgery. J Avian Med Surg 2007;21(1):22–37.
3. Hernandez-Divers SJ, Hernandez-Divers SM, Wilson GH, et al. A review of reptile diagnostic coelioscopy. J Herp Med Surg 2005;15(3):16–31.
4. Innis C, Hernandez-Divers SJ, Martinez-Jimenez D. Coelioscopic-assisted pre-femoral oophorectomy in chelonians. J Am Vet Med Assoc 2007;230(7): 1049–52.
5. Kehlet H. Surgical stress response: does endoscopic surgery confer an advantage? World J Surg 1999;23(8):801–7.
6. Lagares-Garcia JA, Bansidhar B, Moore RA. Benefits of laparoscopy in middle-aged patients. Surg Endosc 2003;17(1):68–72.
7. Innis CJ. Innovative approaches to chelonian obstetrics. Exotic DVM 2004;6(3): 78–82.
8. Knotek Z, Jekl V, Knotkova Z, et al. Eggs in chelonian urinary bladder: is coeliotomy necessary? In: Proceedings of the Association of Reptilian and Amphibian Veterinarians Sixteenth Annual Conference. Milwaukee (WI), August 8–15, 2009. p. 118–21.
9. Innis CJ, Boyer TH. Chelonian reproductive disorders. Vet Clin North Am Exot Anim Pract 2002;5(3):555–78.
10. Keymer IF. Diseases of chelonians: (1) necropsy survey of tortoises. Vet Rec 1978;103(25):548–52.
11. Keymer IF. Diseases of chelonians: (2) necropsy survey of terrapins and turtles. Vet Rec 1978;103(26–7):577–82.
12. McArthur S. Follicular stasis in captive chelonia, *Testudo* spp. In: Proceedings of the Association of Reptilian and Amphibian Veterinarians Eighth Annual Conference. Orlando (FL), September 19–23, 2001. p. 75–86.
13. Nutter FB, Lee DD, Stamper MA, et al. Hemiovariosalpingectomy in a loggerhead sea turtle (*Caretta caretta*). Vet Rec 2000;146(3):78–80.
14. Jekl V, Hauptman K, Knotek Z. Cloacoscopy in chelonians–a valuable diagnostic tool for reproductive tract evaluation. In: Proceedings of the 43rd International Symposium on Diseases of Zoo and Wild Animals. Edinburgh (UK), May 16–20, 2007. p. 162–3.
15. Thomas HL, Willer CJ, Wosar MA, et al. Egg-retention in the urinary bladder of a Florida cooter turtle, *Pseudemys floridana floridana*. J Herp Med Surg 2002; 11(4):4–6.
16. Boulon RH, Dutton PH, McDonald DL. Leatherback sea turtles (*Dermochelys coriacea*) on St. Croix, U.S. Virgin Islands: fifteen years of conservation. Chelonian Conservation and Biology 1996;2(2):141–7.
17. Buhlman KA, Lynch TK, Gibbons JW. Prolonged egg retention in the turtle *Deirochelys reticularia* in South Carolina. Herpetologica 1995;51(4):457–62.
18. Mader DR, Bennett RA, Funk RS, et al. Surgery. In: Mader DR, editor. Reptile medicine and surgery. 2nd edition. St. Louis (MO): Elsevier; 2006. p. 581–630.
19. Jaeger G, Wosar M, Harms C, et al. Use of a supraplastron approach to the coelomic cavity for repair of an esophageal tear in a loggerhead sea turtle. J Am Vet Med Assoc 2003;223(3):353–5.
20. Brannian RE. A soft tissue laparotomy technique in turtles. J Am Vet Med Assoc 1984;185(11):1416–7.

21. Gould WJ, Yaegar AE, Glennon JC. Surgical correction of an intestinal obstruction in a turtle. J Am Vet Med Assoc 1992;200(5):705–6.
22. Di Bello A, Valastro C, Staffieri F. Surgical approach to the coelomic cavity through the axillary and inguinal regions in sea turtles. J Am Vet Med Assoc 2006;228(6):922–5.
23. Rostal D, Grumbles J, Lance V, et al. Non-lethal sexing techniques for hatchling and immature desert tortoises (*Gopherus agassizii*). Herpetological Monographs 1994;8:103–16.
24. Hernandez-Divers SJ, Stahl S, Farrell R. An endoscopic method for identifying sex of hatchling Chinese box turtles and comparison of general versus local anesthesia for laparoscopy. J Am Vet Med Assoc 2009;234(6):800–4.
25. Stahl SJ. Cloacal endoscopy and associated endosurgical techniques in snakes. In: Proceedings of the Association of Reptilian and Amphibian Veterinarians 12th Annual Conference. Tucson (AZ), April 10–14, 2005. p. 44–6.

Exotic Mammal Diagnostic Endoscopy and Endosurgery

Stephen J. Divers, BVetMed, DZooMed, DACZM, DipECZM(herp), FRCVS

KEYWORDS

- Rabbit • Rodent • Ferret • Exotic mammal
- Minimally invasive • Surgery • Endoscopy

With more than 10 million pet rabbits (*Oryctolagus cuniculus*), ferrets (*Mustela putorius furo*), and rodents (order Rodentia) in the United States, these exotic mammals represent the third largest group of companion mammals (behind dogs and cats).[1] This group represents an expanding component of small animal practice, with many clients expecting the same level of medicine for them compared with our more traditional clientele. The advent of the Association of Exotic Mammal Veterinarians, the American Board of Veterinary Practitioner Board in exotic companion mammals, and the American College of Zoological Medicine Day 2 certifying examination in zoologic companion species have further galvanized the need for veterinarians to provide the expected high quality care being demanded for these species. The majority of rabbits, ferrets, and rodents presented to practitioners are less than 2 kg, and given their small size, they are ideal candidates for minimally invasive diagnostic and surgical endoscopy. Indeed, in some situations the development of endoscopy has enabled many procedures to be performed for the first time or with significantly reduced morbidity and mortality compared with traditional surgery. Considerable advances in exotic animal endoscopy have been made over the past 5 years, and further development and refinement seems assured.[2]

PATIENT SELECTION

Unlike ferrets (Carnivora), rabbits and rodents are prey animals and as such will generally mask symptoms until disease is advanced. Consequently, many rabbits and rodents may require improved preanesthetic nursing support (particularly analgesic, fluid therapy, and nutrition) before anesthesia and endoscopy.

The most common endoscopic procedures performed in rabbits and rodents are stomatoscopy (examination of the oral cavity), rhinoscopy, otoscopy, cystoscopy,

Department of Small Animal Medicine & Surgery (Zoological Medicine), College of Veterinary Medicine, University of Georgia, 501 DW Brooks Drive, Athens, GA 30602, USA
E-mail address: sdivers@uga.edu

Vet Clin Exot Anim 13 (2010) 255–272
doi:10.1016/j.cvex.2010.01.006
1094-9194/10/$ – see front matter © 2010 Elsevier Inc. All rights reserved.

laparoscopy, and as an aid to endotracheal intubation. In ferrets, laparoscopy and gastroscopy are probably most common. In addition to anesthetic contraindications, obesity can hamper laparoscopy, but in most cases it is small patient size that presents the greatest challenge to the exotic mammal endoscopist.

PATIENT EVALUATION

Detailed husbandry and medical anamneses are essential because many ailments are associated with poor captive management. Ideally, hematology, plasma biochemistry, and urinalysis should precede anesthesia. However, in many cases short-term anesthesia may be required for the collection of such samples; whereas, in small rodents the required volume may prove difficult to obtain. In addition, regional survey radiographs are advised before endoscopy.

ANESTHESIA

The diversity within exotic mammal taxa necessitates generalities rather than specifics, and reference should be made to the extensive literature on rabbit, ferret, rodent, small primate, and insectivore anesthesia for precise drug dosages.[3–5] Ferrets are typically fasted for 6 to 8 hours. Rabbits and rodents seldom vomit or regurgitate, and are fasted (which includes removal of food and all bedding materials) for only 1 to 2 hours to reduce material within the oral cavity. An opioid-benzodiazepine premedicant is generally effective and, following preoxygenation by mask, induction can be accomplished using intravenous or intramuscular ketamine alone or in combination with additional benzodiazepine (rabbits and rodents), or intravenous propofol (ferrets). Unlike ferrets in which it is easy to place an endotracheal tube, rabbits and rodents are more challenging, and (unlike gas induction) ketamine provides more time for visualization, application of local anesthetic, and careful visual intubation. Further details on intubation are covered by Johnson elsewhere in this issue. Small rodents that cannot be intubated are best induced and maintained using isoflurane or sevoflurane with oxygen via a close fitting rodent mask and dedicated non-rebreathing rodent circuit. Animals are maintained on isoflurane or sevoflurane in oxygen adjusted to individual patient requirements. Ventilation is often required, especially in rabbits and rodents in dorsal recumbency because of their small thoracic volumes combined with increased gastrointestinal pressure on their diaphragm, thereby reducing spontaneous tidal volume. Ventilation is essential for laparoscopy, thoracoscopy, and when using neuromuscular blockade (eg, rhinoscopy). Hypothermia is difficult to prevent unless warm water or air circulating blankets, and drapes or covers are used. Warming air filters attached to the endotracheal tube can also be useful for maintaining temperature but often require ventilator support in small animals. In addition to reflexes and muscle tone, anesthesia monitoring should include temperature, pulse, respiratory rate, end-tidal capnography, pulse oximetry, and direct or indirect blood pressure. Many of these aids become increasing problematic as animal size decreases. During rhinoscopy of rabbits and larger rodents, intranasal lidocaine and short-term neuromuscular blockade using atracurium further enhances immobilization that would otherwise require a much deeper plane of general anesthesia.

Intraoperative fluid support is important and can be delivered through intravenous (aural, cephalic, saphenous, or jugular) or intraosseous (femoral, humeral) catheters using syringe drivers. In cases where catheterization is not possible, fluids can be administered subcutaneously in the scruff immediately following induction and again on recovery. After extubation, small mammals should be provided oxygen via a loose mask until fully conscious, and then returned to a warm incubator until normothermic. Postoperative fluids, nutrition, and analgesia are essential for rapid recovery and return to normal function.

INSTRUMENTATION

Given the variation in size and the nature of the procedures that may be performed, a variety of different scopes and instruments may be required. For most practices the 2.7 mm system offers the greatest versatility, which can be built upon as individual practice caseload dictates. This system offers several advantages including single-entry procedures, ports for air or saline infusion, and an operating channel for the introduction of 1.7 mm instruments. In addition, the 1.9 mm telescope with integrated sheath and the 1 mm semi-rigid miniscope are extremely useful for smaller mammals. For multiple-entry endoscopy, the recent application of human pediatric 2 and 3 mm instruments to exotic animal endoscopy has enabled laparoscopy and thoracoscopy

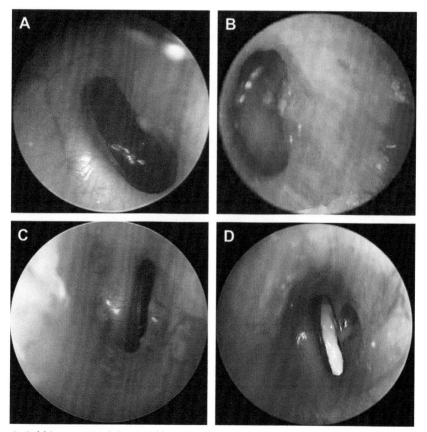

Fig. 1. Rabbit otoscopy. (*A*) Normal horizontal canal and tympanum. (*B*) Inflamed horizontal canal with caseous debris visible behind an intact tympanum. (*C*) Ruptured tympanum without evidence of inflammation or infection. (*D*) Otitis media with ruptured tympanum and caseous debris visible. (*Courtesy of* Stephen J. Divers, Athens, GA.)

to become a reality.[6] For more detailed information see the article that discusses equipment and instrumentation elsewhere in this issue.

PROCEDURES

In general, the approach to exotic mammal endoscopy is similar to domesticated dogs and cats, and much can be learned and applied from the domestic animal and human literature.[7,8] However, in addition to the anatomic peculiarities, the exotic mammal endoscopist must be more precise given the confines within these species. It is therefore particularly important to use finger and thumb of the inferior hand to support the tip of the telescope to ensure accurate control at all times.

Otoscopy

With the anesthetized animal in sternal or lateral recumbency, a detailed evaluation of the ears can be undertaken. In cases of severe disease, superficial exudates and debris should be gently removed before employing sterile saline infusion and working within a fluid environment. Abnormalities can be sampled for histopathology and microbiology using the biopsy forceps, which tend to provide more precise results than introducing a culturette down the vertical canal. Depending upon the size of the animal, diameter of the scope, and nature of the aural disease, it is often possible to examine the vertical and horizontal canals down to the tympanum (**Fig. 1**). It is especially important to examine the tympanum in rabbits and rodents because head tilt caused by otitis media or interna is common. In ferrets, ear mites and aural neoplasia appear to be more common than bacterial infection.

Stomatoscopy

Dental disease is undoubtedly one of the most common presentations for rabbits and rodents, and stomatoscopy under general anesthesia ensures a far more detailed examination than can be achieved in the conscious animal in the examination

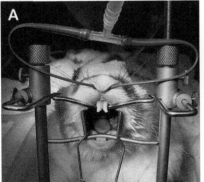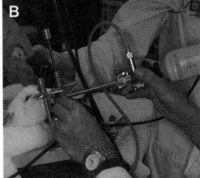

Fig. 2. Rabbit stomatoscopy. (*A*) Positioning of an anesthetized rabbit for intraoral endoscopy using a dental rack, cheek dilators, and nasal oxygen. This system allows positional versatility for a variety of small exotic mammals. (*B*) Positioning of the telescope and light guide cable to capitalize on the 30° viewing angle for examination of the mandibular teeth. Rotating the telescope 180° around its longitudinal axis (such that the light guide cable faces down) facilitates examination of the maxillary teeth. In this case the rabbit is being maintained via a small nasal cone. (*Courtesy of* Stephen J. Divers, Athens, GA.)

room.[2,9,10] The limited access to the oral cavity may preclude the use of endotracheal tubes; however, anesthetic gas and oxygen can be supplied via nasal intubation or by placing a small face mask over the nostrils. It is important to give consideration to the use of active scavenging from the area to avoid anesthetic gas exposure to staff. Alternatively, injectable anesthetic agents may be used, and although this does not negate the need for supplying oxygen via nasal line or mask, it does reduce staff exposure to inhalant agents. The animal is positioned in sternal recumbency with the head supported and mouth held open using a rodent/rabbit table retractor restrainer and cheek spreaders (Sontec Instruments Inc., Centennial, CO 80112, USA). The 1.9 or 2.7 mm telescope are preferred because the 30° angle provides a better view of the occlusal

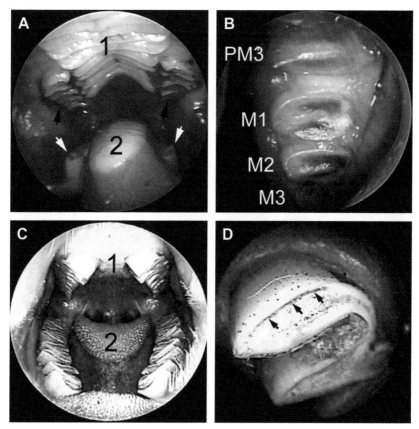

Fig. 3. Intraoral endoscopy in a normal rabbit and guinea pig. (*A*) General overview of the oral cavity of a normal rabbit. The hard palate (1) and tongue (2) are labeled for orientation, and note that the maxillary crowns (*black arrows*) are naturally shorter than the mandibular crowns (*white arrows*). (*B*) Normal left maxillary arcade in a rabbit demonstrating the third premolar (PM3), and the first, second, and third molar teeth (M1–3). (*C*) General overview of the oral cavity of a normal guinea pig. The hard palate (1) and tongue (2) are labeled for orientation, and note the angular slope of the dental arcades when compared with the rabbit. (*D*) Close-up of a maxillary molar in a guinea pig demonstrating the enamel-dentine interface (*arrows*) that produces the cusps that aid forage mastication. (*Courtesy of* Stephen J. Divers, Athens, GA.)

surfaces; with the light guide cable down the view is angled toward the maxillary arcades, and with the light guide cable up the mandibular teeth are preferentially seen (**Fig. 2**). The lingual, buccal, and occlusal aspects of every tooth should be evaluated using appropriately sized and curved dental probes. Tooth laxity, exudates, and gingival changes should be noted. In the vast majority of the small herbivores, the most commonly encountered malocclusions involve overgrowth to the lingual aspect of the lower arcades and buccal aspect of the upper arcades (**Figs. 3** and **4**). Once identified, the malocclusion should be trimmed with rongeurs, a dental rasp, or preferably a motorized dental hand piece that is less likely to result in dental fracture (**Fig 5**). During dental trimming it is vital that the telescope is either protected using a guard, or temporarily removed and later reinserted to evaluate the teeth following reduction of the malocclusion. The telescope can also be used periodically to evaluate the intraoperative progress of premolar or molar extractions or to examine the cavity left following extraction. Indeed, the telescope has also been used to target flushing and antimicrobials into dental cavities via the oral cavity (see **Fig. 5**). These techniques have been used to successfully treat retrobulbar abscesses in rabbits via the oral

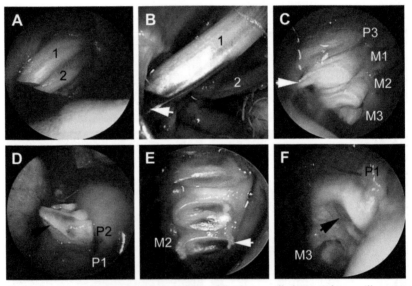

Fig. 4. Endoscopic dental pathology in rabbits. (*A*) Abnormally long right maxillary premolars 1 and 2 caused by inadequate dietary forage. (*B*) Close-up of more severe elongation of the right maxillary premolars 1 and 2. In this case the teeth have caused severe ulceration in the buccal mucosa (*arrow*). (*C*) Mild elongation of right maxillary premolar 3, molar 1, and molar 2; molar 3 appears normal. Note that molar 1 also has a small sharp spur associated with its buccal border (*arrow*). This spur would be buried in the buccal mucosa and would be impossible to visualize without endoscopy and lateral retraction of the mucosa. (*D*) Gross elongation of left mandibular premolar 2 with associated lingual spur (*arrow*), and fracture or severe wear of premolar 1 to the level of the gingival. (*E*) Caseous exudate emanating from around the left maxillary molar 2 following the application of pressure using a dental probe. (*F*) End stage dental disease. In this view of the left maxillary arcade only premolar 1 and molar 3 are clearly visible, premolar 2 and molar 2 are missing, whereas part of molar 1 (*arrow*) can be seen emerging from swollen gingiva that may well indicate an underlying dental abscess. (*Courtesy of* Stephen J. Divers, Athens, GA.)

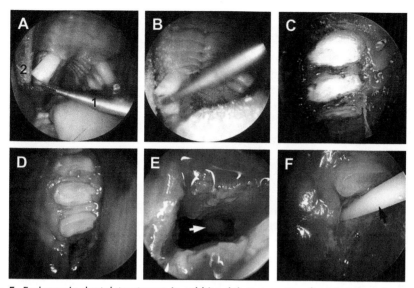

Fig. 5. Endoscopic dental treatment in rabbits. (*A*) Preparation for trimming elongated maxillary premolars and molars using a dental burr (1). Note the metal probe (2) being used to retract and protect the buccal mucosa from the burr. (*B*) High-speed dental burring requires great care to protect the soft tissues and the telescope. Metal probes and guards should always be used. (*C*) Immediate postoperative view of the maxillary arcade following burring down to the level of the gingival. (*D*) Immediate postoperative view following intraoral extraction of molars 2 and 3 causing a retrobulbar abscess. (*E*) Close-up of the extraction site demonstrating the ability of the 30° telescope to look into the abscess cavity and visualize the maxillary bone (*arrow*). (*F*) Placement of an intravenous catheter (*arrow*) into the abscess cavity to instill antibiotic-impregnated synthetic bioactive ceramic material. (*Courtesy of* Stephen J. Divers, Athens, GA.)

cavity, thereby avoiding enucleation.[11] Although rare, soft-tissue masses may be biopsied using the 1.7 mm biopsy forceps, whereas foreign bodies may be removed using retrieval forceps.

Endotracheal Intubation

Intubation is more difficult in rodents and rabbits, and the endoscope can serve as a useful aid for intubation before any prolonged diagnostic or surgical procedure. The endoscope can be used as a laryngoscope to provide visualization of the glottis to aid direct intubation. The author favors inserting the endoscope into the endotracheal tube, passing the endoscope through the glottis, and then advancing the tube off the endoscope and into the trachea (**Fig. 6**). See the article by Johnson elsewhere in this issue for more detailed information on this topic.

Tracheobronchoscopy

Small flexible bronchoscopes can be used to examine the trachea and bronchi on larger rabbits and rodents; however, small telescopes can also be used to gain access to the level of the tracheal bifurcation and beyond (**Fig. 7**). It is vital that on entering the glottis, the head and neck are kept straight and extended to avoid mucosal damage as

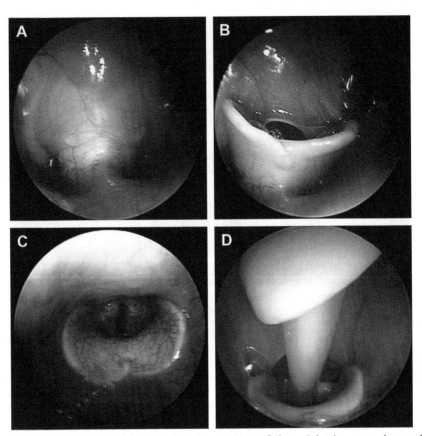

Fig. 6. Rabbit intubation. (*A*) Normal resting position of the epiglottis engaged over the caudal edge of the soft palate in an obligate nasal breathing rabbit. (*B*) Following induction and with the head and neck extended, the endoscope is used to displace the soft palate dorsad to free the epiglottis. (*C*) With the epiglottis now lying ventrad in the oropharynx, the glottis can be clearly seen. (*D*) Following the application of local anesthetic, the endotracheal and stylet are inserted into the trachea. (*Courtesy of* Stephen J. Divers, Athens, GA.)

the telescope is advanced. Unless oxygenation can be maintained, tracheobronchoscopy evaluations are necessarily brief.

Rhinoscopy

With the animal intubated and in sternal recumbency in a 10 to 20° head-down position, the oropharynx is packed with moistened gauze. The nasal cavities are flushed using warm sterile saline to remove any debris and excess mucus from the nasal cavities (**Fig. 8**A). The use of towels under the animals' head helps prevent flooding of the table and floor. For animals more than 2 kg, the 2.7 mm telescope is used, but for smaller animals the 1.9 mm sheathed telescope is preferred (see **Fig. 8**B). Using a sheath enables intraoperative flushing to maintain visualization; however, in small animals the naked telescope can be used with care along with intermittent syringe flushing through the nostrils. The ventral and middle nasal meati can be exploited to

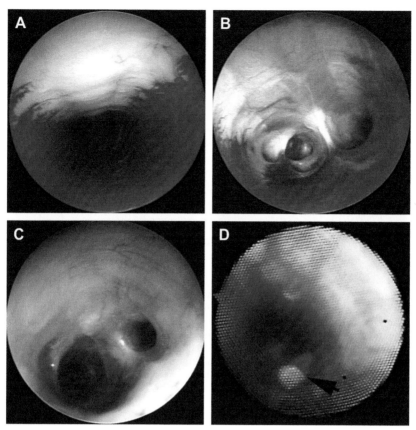

Fig. 7. Rabbit tracheobronchoscopy. Telescopic views of the normal anterior trachea (*A*), bifurcation (*B*), bronchus and secondary bronchi (*C*). (*D*) Flexible endoscopic view of the bifurcation with a foreign body lodged in a primary bronchus (*arrow*). (*Courtesy of* Stephen J. Divers, Athens, GA.)

examine the ventral and middle conchae. In larger animals, the endoturbinates and opening to the nasopharynx can also be seen. Care is required to avoid damaging the delicate nasal turbinates that are prone to hemorrhage (**Fig. 9**A). The telescope should be kept as medial as possible and always kept within the meati. Even so, hemorrhage can rarely be completely avoided. Exudates, abscesses, masses, and foreign bodies can be appreciated and biopsied or removed (see **Fig. 9**B-F).

The recent advent of 2 and 3 mm rigid instruments also permits biopsy and debridement within the nasal or paranasal sinuses via limited surgical access.[6] There are occasions when dental disease requires an extraoral approach, either alone or in conjunction with intraoral surgery, and the telescope can serve as a useful surgical aid. The extension of hypsodont roots into the nasal cavity may warrant rhinoscopy via the nostrils, as detailed earlier, or surgical rhinotomy. Dental abscesses affecting the maxilla may enter the paranasal sinuses and the telescope can provide evaluation via a small (4–5 mm) osteotomy. Even when extensive surgical osteotomy or rhinotomy are performed, surgical access is often limited in small herbivores, but the telescope enables detailed evaluation including those areas cranial and caudal to the surgical site (**Fig. 10**).

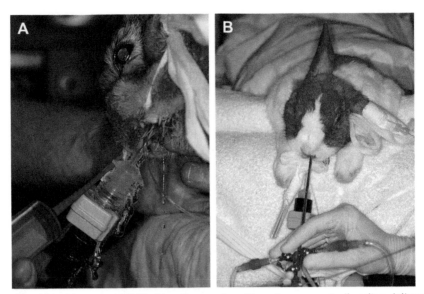

Fig. 8. Rabbit rhinoscopy. (*A*) Flushing the nasal cavities using warm sterile saline delivered using a 60 mL syringe and cut-down 8F red rubber catheter. Packing the oral cavity with gauze and use of a cuffed endotracheal tube are essential. (*B*) Performing rhinoscopy using a 2.7 mm telescope and 4.8 mm operating sheath. A bag of sterile saline suspended above the table is connected to one of the sheath ports by an intravenous administration set and facilitates intraoperative flushing. A second administration set is connected to the second sheath port and provides an egress to a collection bucket under the table. (*Courtesy of Stephen J. Divers, Athens, GA.*)

Vaginoscopy and Cystoscopy

Hematuria is not uncommon in rabbits and rodents, and can be related to diseases affecting the urinary or reproductive systems. With the animal in dorsal recumbency and the perineum close to the table edge, a small 30° sheathed telescope can be inserted through the vulva and into the vagina. Using sterile saline infusion, it is certainly possible to evaluate the vagina, urethra, bladder, and the surface of the cervices of animals as small as 500 g (**Fig. 11**).

Gastroscopy and Colonoscopy

Gastrointestinal disease is especially common in ferrets. However, there has been a noticeable absence of endoscopy in the pursuit of definitive diagnoses, which is unfortunate because ferrets and other small mammals more than 1 kg can often accommodate the smaller flexible gastroscopes, whereas the stomach can often be reached using telescopes in animals less than 1 kg (**Fig. 12**). The ability to confirm the presence of gastric ulceration and collect mucosal biopsies for cultures and histology should be considered routine in the investigation of gastric diseases in ferrets (**Fig. 13**A, B). Unfortunately, the stomach of small herbivores is never empty, which can make endoscopic evaluation near impossible.

Rodent colonoscopy recently became important because researchers were looking for a means of following the progression of human colon cancer in a rodent model. The 1.9 mm sheathed telescope has been used to examine the rectum and descending colon of mice as small as 20 g. The ability to infuse methylene blue and other chemical

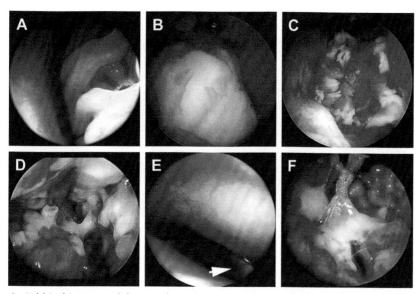

Fig. 9. Rabbit rhinoscopy. (*A*) Normal nasal turbinates viewed from within the ventral nasal meatus. (*B*) Abscess in the caudal aspect of the ventral nasal meatus in a rabbit previously treated for chronic rhinitis. (*C*) Same abscess following endoscopic debridement which with postoperative antimicrobials, based on biopsy culture and sensitivity, were curative. (*D*) Granulomatous rhinitis with nasal septum destruction caused by *Mycobacterium* sp. (*E*) Hay foreign body (*arrow*) within the cranial aspect of the ventral nasal meatus, just caudal to the alar fold. (*F*) Ventral conchal atrophy and chronic rhinitis. (*Courtesy of* Stephen J. Divers, Athens, GA.)

markers via the operating sheath has further improved the ability to identify colonic cells undergoing early neoplastic transformation using so-called chromoendoscopy (see **Fig. 13**C, D).[12] The same system and technique can be employed in companion rodents, with the animal in sternal or lateral recumbency and the perineum close to the table edge.

Laparoscopy

For a detailed discussion of methodology the reader is referred to the dedicated laparoscopy literature, because only small-mammal specifics are highlighted here.[7,8,13] Laparoscopy has been shown to offer significant advantages over traditional surgical options in human and veterinary medicine. In particular, laparoscopy is, with practice, faster, less traumatic, results in less postoperative pain, and faster return to normal function. Until the advent of 2 and 3 mm human pediatric equipment, small mammal laparoscopy was limited to a single-entry system using the sheathed telescope. However, multiple-entry techniques are now possible and practical for animals more than 500 to 1000 g. Indeed, laparoscopic ovariectomy is now the author's sterilization method of choice for female rodents and rabbits because it involves less tissue manipulation and results in less postoperative discomfort and faster return to normal feeding and behavior.

Single-entry laparoscopy has been used most extensively for the collection of visceral biopsies from rodents and rabbits. In general, a 3- to 4-mm surgical approach is made through the umbilicus or at some other convenient point along the linea alba

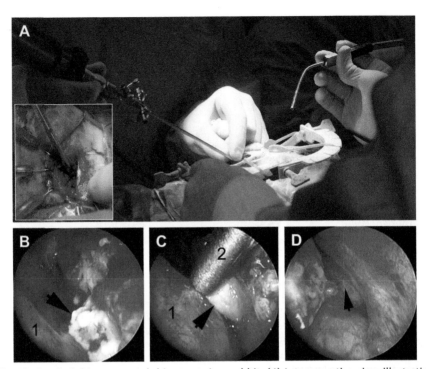

Fig. 10. Surgical rhinotomy and rhinoscopy in a rabbit. (*A*) Intraoperative view illustrating the use of the telescope to examine the nasal cavity following rhinotomy. Insert, close-up of the introduction of the telescope through the rhinotomy. (*B*) Endoscopic view of caseous exudate (*arrow*) within the ventral nasal meatus following the removal of chronically infected turbinates. The nasal septum (1) is labeled for orientation. (*C*) Exposure of an overgrown maxillary tooth (*arrow*) that has extended into the nasal cavity and caused the infection. The nasal septum (1) is labeled for orientation, and the suction probe (2) is also visible. (*D*) Intraoperative view following tooth extraction and flushing of the site, revealing a now clear and unhindered ventral nasal meatus leading to the nasopharynx (*arrow*). (*Courtesy of* Stephen J. Divers, Athens, GA.)

(**Fig. 14**). Following insertion of the sheathed telescope, a mattress suture can be tied to create an air-tight seal; however, this is seldom necessary if the incision through the linea alba is small. For larger rabbits and rodents, CO_2 insufflation is required; however, for small rodents it is often possible to simply attach a syringe containing air to one of the sheath ports and manually inject into the abdomen. Risks associated with air embolism have not been observed in rodents but should be considered. Single-entry techniques are simple and easy to perform, but the variety of instruments is limited and so tissue manipulation and endosurgery are rudimental. Nevertheless, visceral evaluation and biopsy is practical even in small rodents (see **Fig. 14**B–D). For larger animals multiple-entry techniques using 2 and 3 mm human pediatric instruments are preferred and provide greater opportunities for endosurgery.[6] There is a wider equipment selection for 3 mm instruments, which are used with click-line interchangeable handles connected to a radiosurgery unit for hemostasis. Access to the abdomen is achieved using a lightweight 3.5 mm (for instruments) and 3.9 mm

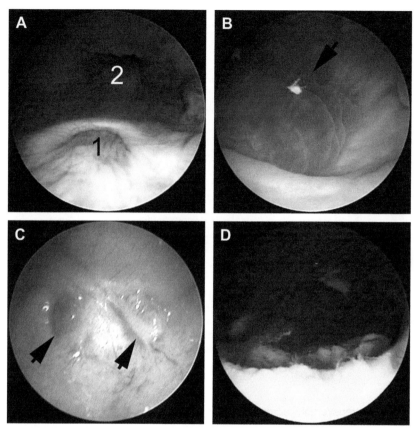

Fig. 11. Rabbit urogenital endoscopy. (*A*) View within the anterior vagina demonstrating the urethra (1) and caudal vaginal vault (2). (*B*) Urethral carcinoma (*arrow*) seen within the anterior vagina. (*C*) Cervices (*arrows*) seen from within the caudal vagina. (*D*) Urinary sand seen within a saline-infused bladder. (*Courtesy of* Stephen J. Divers, Athens, GA.)

(sheathed telescope) threaded graphite cannula. Cannula placement is determined by the organ of interest, preference of the surgeon, and anatomic nature of the animal in question (**Fig. 15**). CO_2 insufflation using a dedicated endoflator is essential for multiple-entry techniques. Some prefer the use of a veress needle, whereas others, concerned about the risk for damage to internal viscera (especially the voluminous gastrointestinal tract of small herbivores), prefer to surgically place the initial cannula or telescope. An ability to rotate the animal from dorsal into either lateral can greatly assist with the location of ovaries, kidneys, and other dorsolateral structures.

For procedures involving dorsolateral structures (eg, ovariectomy), the telescope is inserted through the umbilicus with two additional cannulae placed 2- to 5-cm cranial and caudal to the telescope, along the linea alba. In this way, the instruments can be directed to one lateral. When required to examine the other lateral, the surgeon simply moves around the table. It is often helpful to have a second slave monitor located on the other side of the operating table rather than move the entire endoscopy tower.

For access to the liver, gastrointestinal tract, spleen, pancreas, and bladder, the telescope is again passed through the linea alba or umbilicus, but the instruments

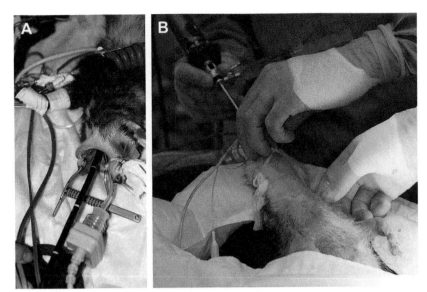

Fig. 12. Ferret gastrointestinal endoscopy. (*A*) Flexible gastroscopy using a 8.6 mm gastro-scope. Such flexible endoscopes provide greater flexibility but are limited to larger mammals (more than 1 to 2 kg). (*B*) Esophagostomy and gastroscopy being performed with a 2.7 mm telescope and sheath with sterile infusion provided by the attached syringe. Such techniques can be used in mammals less than1 kg. (*Courtesy of* Stephen J. Divers, Athens, GA.)

are inserted transversely across the abdomen rather than longitudinally. In this manner, the telescope and instruments can be advanced into the cranial abdomen for access to the liver, stomach and intestinal tract, spleen, and pancreas, or advanced caudally toward the large intestine and bladder (**Fig. 16**). It is important to aspirate all abdominal gas following surgery as the presence of residual gas is a source of postoperative discomfort. Cannula holes are closed using a single suture.

Thoracoscopy

Thoracoscopy remains within its infancy and few clinical applications have been real-ized in rabbits, rodents, or ferrets. Given the recent advances in human pediatric equipment, surgeon ability is probably the major limiting factor, although the small thorax of rodents and rabbits will always present greater challenges. To date, a handful of thoracoscopy procedures have been performed in small mammals. All cases involved evaluation and biopsy of an intrathoracic mass where less invasive ultra-sound-guided fine-needle aspirate cytology proved inconclusive. In all cases, a single-entry system was used with targeted telescope entry based upon preopera-tive imaging. In general, the paraxiphoid approach is easier in most rabbits and rodents less than 2 kg, whereas an intercostal approach is preferred for ferrets and larger rabbits/rodents. Again, the ports are closed using single sutures, and although the placement of a chest drain is not always necessary if all air has been aspirated from the pleural cavity, they should certainly be considered in cases of poor oxygen status and abnormal blood gas values. When such tubes are used, intermittent nega-tive pressure is applied and the tubes are removed once they are nonproductive for more than 30 minutes.

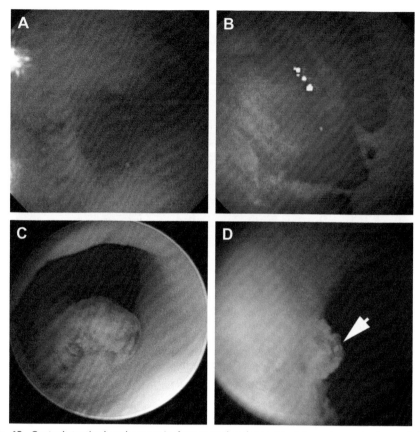

Fig. 13. Gastrointestinal endoscopy in ferrets and rodents. Flexible endoscopic views of the normal gastric mucosa (*A*) and gastric ulceration caused by *Helicobacter mustelae* (*B*) in a ferret. (*C*) Telescopic view of a carcinoma protruding into the lumen of the descending colon in a mouse. (*D*) Early neoplastic transformation in the colon (arrow) can be more easily detected using methylene blue dye. (*Courtesy of* Stephen J. Divers, Athens, GA.)

Complications

The major complications encountered are typically associated with anesthesia and related to issues of debilitation, poor ventilation, lack of vascular access, and hypothermia. The importance of a thorough preoperative evaluation, endotracheal intubation, intravenous or intraosseous catheterization, and warm air/water blankets cannot be over emphasized. Hemorrhage following rhinoscopy or tissue biopsy is common but seldom severe, although it is wise to have hemostatic agents available. Most endoscopy issues are related to operator error until experience and ability have been gained. To facilitate endoscopy caseload without compromising clients or patients, it is recommended that the surgeon retains the option to convert to a traditional surgical approach if required.

POSTOPERATIVE CARE

The immediate postoperative period following extubation is usually the most critical, and oxygen and thermal support should be continued until the animal is fully

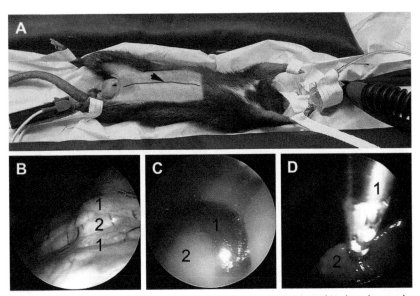

Fig. 14. Single-entry rodent laparoscopy. (*A*) Rat intubated, positioned in dorsal recumbency and prepared for laparoscopy. The linea alba is indicated and the preferred insertion point is the umbilicus (*arrow*). (*B*) View of the right cranial quadrant illustrating the pancreas (1) and duodenum (2) of a guinea pig. (*C*) Normal rabbit kidney (1) partially obscured by retroperitoneal fat (2). Obesity is commonly encountered and complicates laparoscopy. (*D*) Biopsy forceps (1) harvesting a liver, (2) sample from a rat. (*Courtesy of* Stephen J. Divers, Athens, GA.)

conscious and ambulatory. Opioid analgesics may be continued following major procedures; however, nonsteroidal antiinflammatory drugs (eg, meloxicam) are used routinely. Rabbits and rodents are expected to resume feeding within 2 hours, otherwise assisted feeding is initiated and fluid therapy continued. In addition, auscultation of the gastrointestinal tract is routine, with ileus promptly treated using cisapride.

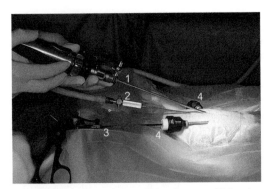

Fig. 15. Multiple-entry laparoscopy in a ferret. The telescope (1) has been inserted through the umbilicus, cranial to the veress needle (2) and CO_2 insufflation line. A 3 mm instrument (3) has been inserted through one of two 3.5 mm cannula (4). (*Courtesy of* Stephen J. Divers, Athens, GA.)

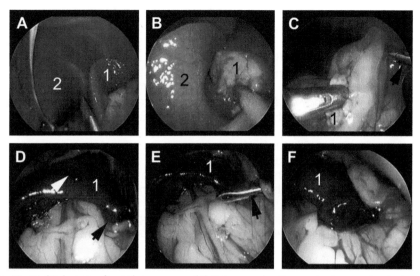

Fig. 16. Multiple-entry ferret laparoscopy. (*A*) Using a palpation probe to examine between the left lateral (*1*) and left medial (*2*) lobes of the liver. (*B*) Identification of an abnormally thickened gall bladder (*1*) between the quadrate and right medial liver lobes (*2*). (*C*) Endoscopic biopsy of the pancreas (*1*) using 3 mm biopsy forceps that confirmed the presence of an insulinoma. Note the use of 3 mm atraumatic tissue forceps (*arrow*) to retract the mesentery. (*D*) View of the spleen (*1*) demonstrating a nodular abnormality (*black arrow*), and the previous site of attempted ultrasound-guided fine-needle aspiration (*white arrow*). (*E*) Biopsy of the spleen (*1*) using 3 mm biopsy forceps (*arrow*). (*F*) Post-biopsy view of the spleen (*1*), note the absence of severe hemorrhage. (*Courtesy of* Stephen J. Divers, Athens, GA.)

OUTCOME

Return to normal behaviors and weight gain are often the most useful indicators for improvement. Clinicopathology can also be useful if abnormalities were detected preoperatively. Serial endoscopic evaluations of the ears, nose, and mouth can be used to monitor patients with otitis, rhinitis, and dental disease.

REFERENCES

1. Avma. U.S. Pet Ownership & Demographics Sourcebook. American Veterinary Medical Association; 2007. Available at: http://www.avma.org/reference/marketstats/ownership.asp. Accessed December 12, 2009.
2. Hernandez-Divers SJ, Murray M. Small mammal endoscopy. In: Quesenberry KE, Carpenter JW, editors. Ferrets, rabbits, and rodents: clinical medicine and surgery. Philadelphia: WB Saunders Co; 2004. p. 392–4.
3. Heard DJ. Lagomorphs (rabbits, hares and pikas). In: West G, Heard D, Caulkett N, editors. Zoo animal & wildlife immobilization and anesthesia. Ames (IA): Blackwell Publishing; 2007. p. 647–53.
4. Heard DJ. Anesthesia, analgesia, and sedation of small mammals. In: Quesenberry KE, Carpenter JW, editors. Ferrets, rabbits, and rodents: clinical medicine and surgery. Philadelphia: WB Saunders Co.; 2004. p. 356–69.
5. Carpenter JW. Exotic animal formulary. 3rd edition. St Louis (MO): WB Saunders Co; 2005.

6. Hernandez-Divers SJ. Minimally-invasive endoscopic surgery of birds. J Avian Med Surg 2005;19(2):107–20.
7. McCarthy TC. Veterinary endoscopy for the small animal practitioner. St Louis (MO): Elsevier; 2005. p. 624.
8. Tams TR. Small animal endoscopy. 2nd edition. St Louis (MO): Mosby; 1999. p. 497.
9. Taylor M. Endoscopy as an aid to the examination and treatment of the oropharyngeal disease of small herbivorous mammals. Semin Avian Exotic Pet Med 1999;8(3):139–41.
10. Hernandez-Divers SJ. Clinical techniques: dental endoscopy of rabbits and rodents. J Exotic Pet Med 2008;17(2):87–92.
11. Martinez-Jimenez D, Hernandez-Divers SJ, Dietrich U, et al. Endosurgical treatment of a retrobulbar abscess in a rabbit. J Am Vet Med Am 2007;230(6): 869–72.
12. Becker C, Fantini MC, Wirtz S, et al. In vivo imaging of colitis and colon cancer development in mice using high resolution chromoendoscopy. Gut 2005;54(7): 950–4.
13. Monnet E, Twedt DC. Laparoscopy. Vet Clin North Am Small Anim Pract 2003; 33(5):1147–63.

Endoscopic Intubation of Exotic Companion Mammals

Dan H. Johnson, DVM

KEYWORDS

- Endoscopy • Intubation • Anesthesia • Trachea
- Airway • Glottis

Tracheal intubation, also referred to as endotracheal intubation, is the placement of a tube into the trachea, usually for the purpose managing a patient's airway during general anesthesia. The term most is often applied to orotracheal intubation, where an endotracheal tube is passed through the mouth, larynx, and vocal cords, into the trachea; nasotracheal intubation and direct intubation through tracheotomy are other possible routes. Tracheal intubation is indicated for the administration of oxygen and inhalant anesthetics, to secure the airway of unconscious patients, and to provide a means of mechanical ventilation. It permits the use of airway monitors; allows a clear surgical approach to the nose, face, and mouth; and also provides a conduit into the trachea for diagnostic, therapeutic, and experimental purposes.[1,2]

The general principles of endotracheal intubation of exotic companion mammals have been thoroughly reviewed.[3–5] Endotracheal intubation provides better airway control during general anesthesia than other methods of airway maintenance (eg, mask or nasal cannula). This is especially important for complex and prolonged procedures, when complications such as respiratory obstruction and hypoventilation are more likely to occur.

Orotracheal intubation of small exotic mammals (particularly rabbits and rodents) is difficult owing to a large tongue, large cheek teeth, small larynx, and a long soft palate that obscures the epiglottis. Many methods have been devised to accomplish orotracheal intubation in exotic companion mammals. Intubation methods are divided into those without visualization of the glottis (blind intubation) and those where the glottis is visualized.[6]

Blind intubation has been described for the rabbit[7–10] and the rat,[11] and it can be applied routinely to other species.[4] By properly positioning the head and neck, the pathway from the oropharynx to the trachea is straightened so that an endotracheal tube can be placed without direct visualization of the larynx. This is possible with the aid of laryngeal palpation, patient response (ie, coughing, gagging), and watching

Avian and Exotic Animal Care, 8711 Fidelity Boulevard, Raleigh, NC 27617, USA
E-mail address: drdan@avianandexotic.com

Vet Clin Exot Anim 13 (2010) 273–289
doi:10.1016/j.cvex.2010.01.010
1094-9194/10/$ – see front matter © 2010 Elsevier Inc. All rights reserved.

for water vapor within the endotracheal tube and listening for patient respiration through it. Under special circumstances, a transtracheally placed wire or catheter may be used as a guide for the endotracheal tube.[12,13]

Orotracheal intubation with visualization of the glottis is the method familiar to most practitioners. Visual intubation methods can be divided further into those that provide either direct visualization or indirect visualization of the glottis.[6] Various methods of direct visual intubation are described for ferrets, rabbits, and rodents.[1,2,4,6,14–20] Direct visualization of the glottis is accomplished best through hyperextension of the head and neck. Usually an assistant positions the patient and holds the mouth open, either with a speculum or with loops of gauze placed around the upper and lower incisors, while the operator uses a small-bladed laryngoscope, otoscope, or other illuminated speculum to depress the tongue and elevate the soft palate. Once the vocal folds are visible, the tube is placed; however, visualization of the glottis usually is lost as the endotracheal tube is placed in the oropharynx.[4,16] Indirect visualization of the trachea can be achieved using an endoscope, video laryngoscope, or video-optical stylet.[21–23] The endoscope or video device is positioned so the larynx is in view, and an endotracheal tube is passed parallel to the instrument and into the trachea. Further, with video-optical stylets and many endoscopes, it is possible to put the instrument directly inside the endotracheal tube and to visually guide the assembly into the trachea. Indirect visualization allows visual confirmation that the endotracheal tube has passed between the vocal cords, and with video-optical stylet and endoscope there is also confirmation that the tube has been placed properly within the tracheal lumen.

Tracheal intubation with indirect visualization is accepted widely in human medicine.[22–27] Indirect visualization has been shown to result in improved intubation success in human infants, even among experienced intubators.[22] Indirect intubation, however, took longer to perform, on average, than direct intubation in emergency room patients.[25] Indirect visualization is the preferred method of intubation for human patients with difficult airway, difficult position, and cervical spinal injury.[22,24,26,28]

Indirect visual intubation also has been documented widely in laboratory animal medicine.[29–34] Veterinary reports of indirect visualization are limited mostly to endoscopic intubation. In each case, endoscopic intubation was documented to be simple, reliable, and safe. The technical challenges posed by rodent and rabbit anatomy were overcome easily, and the success rate for endoscopic intubation approached 100%.[30–33]

Recently, endoscopic intubation has been applied in exotic mammal practice.[21,35–37] Using an endoscope, clinicians are able to intubate mammals ranging in size from rabbits to small rodents. In cases where direct visualization and blind intubation have failed, it is usually possible to intubate the patient with the aid of an endoscope. Intubation of small mammals is difficult to master and requires practice; however, it should be the standard of care for all patients as long as it can be done quickly and safely. Endoscopic intubation provides a versatile, safe, and effective method of endotracheal intubation for exotic companion mammals.

EQUIPMENT

The equipment necessary for endoscopic intubation consists of appropriately sized endotracheal tubes, an endoscope, and a light source.[21,35,38] Most practitioners also use a video camera and video display. Endotracheal tubes either can be commercially obtained or adapted from other materials. The ideal tube size and style vary by species (**Table 1**). Judgment regarding size of a tube can be made based on the

Table 1
Endotracheal tube size/style for selected species

Species	Tube Size	Tube Style
Ferret	2.0–2.5 mm ID	Cole or Murphy
Rabbit	2.0–3.5 mm ID	Cole or Murphy
Prairie dog	2.0–2.5 mm ID	Cole or Murphy
Guinea pig	8 F 2.0–2.5 mm ID	Modified urinary catheter Cole or Murphy
Chinchilla	8 F 0 mm ID	Modified urinary catheter Cole or Murphy
Hedgehog	1.5 mm ID	Straight silicone
Sugar Glider	1.5 mm ID	Straight silicone
Rat	5 mm ID 14 gauge	Straight silicone Intravenous catheter

Abbreviation: ID, internal diameter.

diameter of the laryngeal opening, which, in small mammals, is always smaller than the tracheal lumen.[38] The correct tube will usually be two thirds of the diameter of the tracheal lumen, or roughly the size of the laryngeal opening. To reduce airway resistance, the internal diameter (ID) of the tube selected should be as large as possible (**Table 2**). The author uses two styles of endotracheal tube for most small mammal applications: uncuffed Murphy oral–nasal endotracheal tubes (Sun Med, Largo, FL, USA), sizes 2.0 mm to 3.5 mm (**Fig. 1**); and Cole stepped wall silicone endotracheal tubes (Jorgensen Laboratories, Incorporated, Loveland, CO, USA), sizes 2.0 mm to 3.5 mm (**Fig. 2**). For smaller patients, there are 1.5 and 1.0 mm ID small exotic straight silicone endotracheal tubes (Jorgensen Laboratories, Incorporated), and tubes constructed from intravenous catheters, urinary catheters, and other tubing (**Figs. 3** and **4**). Cuffed endotracheal tubes are appropriate in small mammals, but are difficult to obtain in sizes less than 3.0 mm. Also, a cuff often makes the outer diameter too large for passage through the laryngeal opening (eg, 2.5 mm ID cuffed endotracheal tube has

Table 2
Case example demonstrating how airway resistance increases exponentially as a patient with a 5 mm tracheal lumen is intubated with endotracheal tubes of progressively smaller internal diameter[a]

Tube Size (mm)	Ratio of Endotracheal Tube Internal Diameter to Tracheal Lumen (5 mm)	Increases Airway Resistance by Factor of:
3.5	0.7	5.9
3.0	0.6	12.8
2.5	0.5	32.0
2.0	0.4	97.7

[a] To calculate relative airway resistance, first determine the caliber reduction ratio X; then, relative airway resistance $R = (1/X)^5$. Example: if using a 3 mm tube in a 5 mm trachea, caliber reduction ratio is 3/5 or 0.6, and relative airway resistance equals $(1/0.6)^5$; a 3 mm endotracheal tube increases airway resistance of a 5 mm trachea by a factor of 12.86. (*Data from:* Bock KR, Silver P, Rom M, et al. Reduction in tracheal lumen due to endotracheal intubation and its calculated clinical significance. Chest 2000;118(2):468–73).

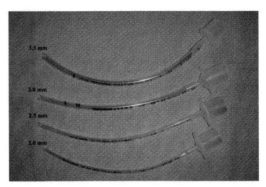

Fig. 1. Uncuffed Murphy oral–nasal endotracheal tubes (Sun Med, Largo, Florida), shown in sizes 3.5 mm to 2.0 mm internal diameter (ID), are familiar to most practitioners. These can be used to intubate patients ranging in size from rabbits to guinea pigs and chinchillas. (*Courtesy of* Dan H. Johnson, DVM, Raleigh, NC.)

an outer diameter of 4.0 mm). Clear endotracheal tubes are preferred in order that water vapor can be observed within the lumen.

Currently, three types of endoscope are widely reported for endotracheal intubation in small exotic mammals: the 2.7 mm 30° Hopkins rod-lens telescope (Karl Storz Veterinary Endoscopy America, Goleta, CA, USA) (**Fig. 5**), the 1.9 mm semirigid fiber optic endoscope (MDS Incorporated, Brandon, FL, USA), and 1.0 mm semirigid fiber optic endoscopes by Karl Storz and MDS (**Fig. 6**). When used for over-the-endoscope intubation, the 2.7 mm telescope can accommodate endotracheal tubes with an internal diameter of 3.0 mm or greater. The 30° angle of the Hopkins telescope permits a clear view of the glottis over the base of the tongue, whereas the 0° angle of the semirigid fiber optic scope does not (**Fig. 7**). The telescope, however, is rigid and vulnerable to damage without its protective sheath. It should not be bent or flexed, which limits its effectiveness in patients with difficult airway or position. With a large field of view, 30° angle, and superior optics, the 2.7 mm rigid endoscope is ideal for side-by-side intubation (**Fig. 8**).

The 1.0 mm and 1.9 mm semi-rigid endoscopes are fiber optic with a metal sheath. They are rigid enough to push the soft palate and to direct the endotracheal tube, yet able to flex without being damaged (**Fig. 9**). Because they are semirigid, the fiber optic endoscopes depend less on patient positioning and are ideal for over-the-endoscope intubation, which typically can be performed by one person (**Fig. 10**). The 1.9 mm

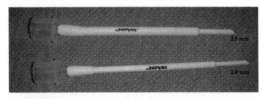

Fig. 2. Cole stepped wall silicone endotracheal tubes (Jorgensen Laboratories, Incorporated, Loveland, Colorado); sizes 2.5 mm and 2.0 mm are pictured. When properly positioned, the glottis forms a seal where the narrow intratracheal segment joins the wider segment. The narrow intratracheal segment is short, which reduces airway resistance when compared with tubes of uniform diameter. (*Courtesy of* Dan H. Johnson, DVM, Raleigh, NC.)

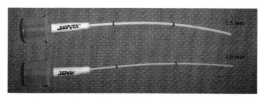

Fig. 3. Small exotic straight silicone endotracheal tubes (Jorgensen Laboratories, Incorporated), 1.5 and 1.0 mm ID, for use in smaller patients. These long, narrow tubes produce maximal airway resistance and are prone to obstruction by respiratory secretions. These tubes may be shortened to minimize airway resistance and better fit the individual patient. (*Courtesy of* Dan H. Johnson, DVM, Raleigh, NC.)

semirigid scope can accommodate endotracheal tubes down to 2.0 mm for over-the-endoscope intubation, and the 1.0 mm semirigid scope accommodate a 1.5 mm endotracheal tube. Both are also suitable for side-by-side intubation; however, the smaller size and fiber optics give the semirigid endoscopes a lower-quality image than the Hopkins rod lens telescope (**Fig. 11**).

Light for endoscopic intubation usually is provided by a tabletop light source and conveyed to the endoscope by a fiber optic light guide cable. Endoscopic intubation also may be performed with the aid of a camera and video monitor. Various interchangeable light source, video camera, and video display options are available for all of these endoscopes. For portability and simplicity, the author prefers to intubate by looking directly through the scope and using a handheld light source (see **Figs. 6** and **10**).[35]

PREPARATION AND GENERAL PROCEDURE

The patient must be sufficiently induced and relaxed to proceed with intubation. The induction window needs to mirror the skill level of the operator. Mask induction with inhalant gas only allows a short time in which to intubate a patient; therefore, single or combination injectable anesthesia is recommended.[37,38] During intubation, it is possible to provide supplemental anesthetic gas via a nasal mask in rabbits and rodents, because they are obligate nasal breathers.[39] Atropine or glycopyrrolate may be indicated to decrease salivary secretions, especially in guinea pigs, which tend to exhibit profuse hypersalivation with inhalant anesthesia.

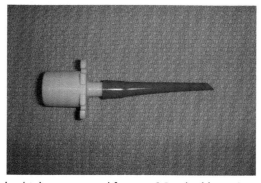

Fig. 4. An endotracheal tube constructed from an 8 F red rubber urinary catheter. Endotracheal tubes can be constructed from intravenous catheters, feeding tubes, and similar items. (*Courtesy of* Dan H. Johnson, DVM, Raleigh, NC.)

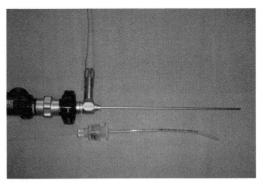

Fig. 5. A 2.7 mm 30° Hopkins rod-lens telescope (Karl Storz Veterinary Endoscopy America, Goleta, California) and 2.5 mm Murphy endotracheal tube; a malleable stylet (Jorgensen Laboratories, Incorporated) has been inserted into the tube to provide rigidity. The endoscope is shown with video camera and light guide cable attached, but without its protective sheath. This scope has a 30° angle tip that gives an excellent view of the glottis, and rod-lens optics for superior image quality (see **Figs. 7** and **11**). (*Courtesy of* Dan H. Johnson, DVM, Raleigh, NC.)

The patient is positioned in sternal or dorsal recumbency with the mouth held open by a mouth gag (**Figs. 12** and **13**). In some cases, an adjustable platform is used to facilitate intubation (see **Fig. 8**).[14,19,20,34] The oral cavity is examined for food or fecal matter and swabbed clean, if necessary. An appropriately sized endotracheal tube is selected (see **Table 1**). By palpating the larynx, the distance to insert the endotracheal tube is premeasured and noted. To reduce laryngospasm and gagging, a small amount of lidocaine injectable solution or viscous lidocaine jelly may be applied to the larynx or the tube tip, respectively.

SIDE-BY-SIDE INTUBATION

The endoscope is advanced over the base of the tongue until the tip of the epiglottis is visible through the soft palate (**Fig. 14**). The tip of the scope is advanced gently in a dorsocaudal direction, lifting the soft palate and thus allowing the epiglottis to fall forward.

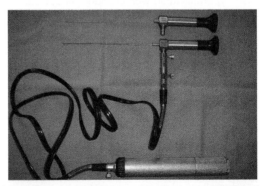

Fig. 6. 1.9 mm and 1.0 mm semirigid fiber optic endoscopes (MDS Incorporated, Brandon, Florida). The 1.9 mm scope is shown with its portable light source attached. Both endoscopes can be fitted for use with the Storz video endoscopy system. (*Courtesy of* Dan H. Johnson, DVM, Raleigh, NC.)

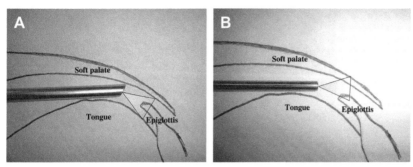

Fig. 7. (*A*) The 30° angle of the Hopkins telescope permits a clear view of the glottis over the base of the tongue, whereas (*B*) the 0° angle of the semirigid fiber optic scope does not. (*Courtesy of* Dan H. Johnson, DVM, Raleigh, NC.)

The scope is withdrawn slightly to visualize the glottis, and positioned off to one side of the epiglottis. An endotracheal tube is introduced into the oral cavity and advanced along the dorsal surface of the tongue until it comes into view. The tip of the tube is placed on the epiglottis and then passed through the glottal opening upon inhalation (see **Fig. 8**). The endoscope allows the operator a clear view of the endotracheal tube as it passes into the trachea. If a stylet was used to introduce the endotracheal tube, it is withdrawn. Through the endoscope, it may be possible to see water vapor in the tube with each breath, providing further evidence of proper placement.

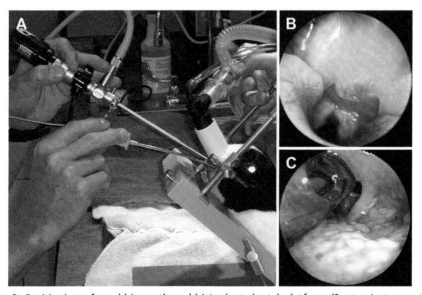

Fig. 8. Positioning of a rabbit on the rabbit/rodent dental platform (Sontec Instruments, Centennial, Colorado) for side-by-side endoscopic tracheal intubation with the 2.7 mm 30° Hopkins rod-lens telescope (Karl Storz Veterinary Endoscopy America), in its protective sheath, with video camera attached (*A*). Endoscopic view through the 2.7 mm 30° telescope of a rabbit glottis during side-by-side intubation using a 2.5 mm Cole endotracheal tube (*B*). Endoscopic view of same in a guinea pig using a 2.0 mm Murphy endotracheal tube and malleable stylet (*C*). (*Courtesy of* Dan H. Johnson, DVM, Raleigh, NC.)

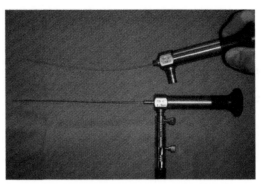

Fig. 9. The 1.0 mm and 1.9 mm semirigid endoscopes are fiber optic with a metal sheath. They are rigid enough to push the soft palate and to direct the endotracheal tube, yet able to flex without being damaged. (*Courtesy of* Dan H. Johnson, DVM, Raleigh, NC.)

OVER-THE-ENDOSCOPE INTUBATION

The endoscope is inserted into an endotracheal tube from its adapter end, and the tip of the scope is positioned to within 1 to 2 mm of the beveled end of the tube, providing a maximal field of view while protecting the patient from the tip of the scope. This position also enables the operator to remove moisture accumulation from the tip of the scope by touching it against oral cavity membranes; if the tip of the scope is positioned too far from the end of the tube, mucous and saliva will collect inside the tip of the endotracheal tube and obscure the operator's view. The endotracheal tube may need to be trimmed at its adapter end to shorten it for this purpose. The endoscope acts as a stylet for the endotracheal tube. The endoscope/endotracheal tube combination is advanced over the base of the tongue until the tip of the epiglottis is visible through the soft palate. The tip of the scope is advanced gently in a dorsocaudal direction, lifting the soft palate and thus allowing the epiglottis to fall forward (see **Fig. 14**). The scope is withdrawn slightly and the endoscope tip is rested on the epiglottis. The glottis is visualized. The tube/scope combination is advanced into the laryngeal opening and into the trachea upon inspiration, where positioning is

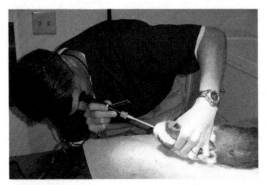

Fig. 10. With a semirigid fiber optic endoscope, over-the-endoscope intubation is less dependent on patient positioning and can be performed by one person. (*Courtesy of* Dan H. Johnson, DVM, Raleigh, NC.)

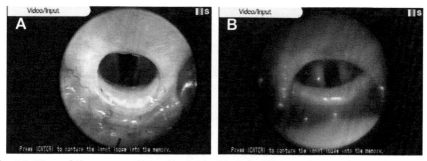

Fig. 11. View of the same guinea pig glottis through a 2.7 mm 30° Hopkins rod-lens tele-scope (*A*) and a 1.9 mm fiber optic endoscope (*B*). The image through the 2.7 rod-lens scope is larger and clearer than that of the 1.9 mm fiber optic endoscope, because of the larger superior optics of the telescope and the mosaic pattern created by the optical fibers within the endoscope. (*Courtesy of* Dan H. Johnson, DVM, Raleigh, NC.)

confirmed by the presence of tracheal rings. The endotracheal tube is advanced off the scope and secured.

COMMENTS ON PARTICULAR SPECIES
Ferret

While direct placement of an endotracheal tube in ferrets (*Mustela furo* [formerly *Mustela putorius furo*]) is relatively simple, it usually requires two people. The jaw tone of ferrets often remains high even at moderate levels of anesthesia; therefore one person must hold the jaws apart while the other pulls the tongue forward and places the tube. Over-the-endoscope intubation of ferrets simplifies intubation, because it does not require the jaws to be opened wide or the tongue to be pulled forward. The endo-scope/tube combination is rigid enough to force the tongue forward at its base, exposing the glottis. The tube and scope are advanced over the epiglottis and into the trachea. The 1.0 mm or 1.9 mm semirigid endoscope with a 2.0 mm to 2.5 mm Cole or uncuffed Murphy endotracheal tube is recommended for intubating ferrets with this technique.

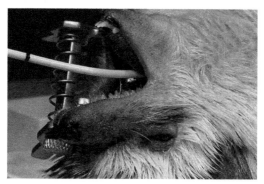

Fig. 12. Spring-loaded Nazzy ferret gag (Jorgensen Laboratories, Incorporated) is suitable for ferrets, hedgehogs, and other small mammals. (*Courtesy of* Dan H. Johnson, DVM, Raleigh, NC.)

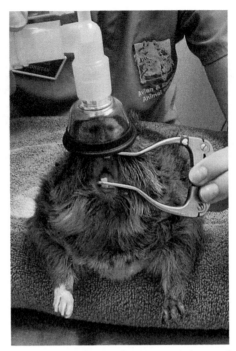

Fig. 13. Positioning of rodent mouth gag (Jorgensen Laboratories, Incorporated) and nasal gas anesthesia for intubation of a guinea pig. (*Courtesy of* Dan H. Johnson, DVM, Raleigh, NC.)

Rabbit

Intubating rabbits (*Oryctolagus cuniculi*) can be a challenge. Many reports emphasize that rabbits are prone to laryngospasm and bronchospasm; however, in the author's experience, these concerns are exaggerated and likely the result of repeated attempts by inexperienced operators. Endoscopic intubation avoids this by providing the intubator a clear view of the objective. Both side-by-side and over-the-endoscope intubation are reported in rabbits. The author prefers over-the-endoscope intubation using the 1.9 mm semirigid scope and 2.0 mm to 3.5 mm uncuffed Murphy or Cole endotracheal tubes.

Prairie Dog

Prairie dogs (*Cynomys ludovicianus*) are intubated in a manner similar to that described for rabbits. They are generally more difficult to intubate, as the glottal opening is slightly smaller than in rabbits. The soft palate of the prairie dog appears to be longer and under less tension than in the rabbit, and it is more difficult to keep the soft palate from obscuring the glottis (see **Fig. 14**). The author prefers to use the over-the-endoscope method with a 2.0 mm to 2.5 mm uncuffed Murphy or Cole endotracheal tube over a semirigid scope.

Guinea Pig/Chinchilla

Guinea pigs (*Cavia porcellus*) and chinchillas (*Chinchilla lanigera*) are generally harder to intubate than the species discussed previously. Guinea pigs and, to a lesser extent, chinchillas, have a narrow palatial ostium formed by the soft palate, palatoglossal

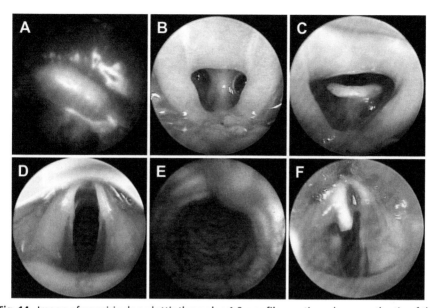

Fig. 14. Image of a prairie dog glottis through a 1.9 mm fiber optic endoscope: the tip of the epiglottis is visible through the soft palate (*A*). View of the guinea pig glottis through the 2.7 mm 30° Hopkins rod-lens telescope (*B through D*). Before disturbing the glottis with the tip of the scope, note the palatial ostium formed by the soft palate dorsally, the palatoglossal arches laterally, and the base of the tongue ventrally (*B*). After displacing the soft palate and allowing the epiglottis to fall forward, bringing the vocal cords into view (*C*). View of the vocal cords and tracheal opening as the tip of the endoscope is advanced over the edge of the epiglottis (*D*). View of a prairie dog tracheal lumen through a 1.9 mm fiber optic scope during over-the-endoscope intubation: proper positioning of the endotracheal tube is confirmed by the presence of tracheal rings and/or bifurcation (*E*). Excessive force during intubation can cause trauma to the glottis or trachea, and may result in injury, edema, or stenosis (*F*). (*Courtesy of* Dan H. Johnson, DVM, Raleigh, NC.)

arches, and tongue (see **Fig. 14**). In addition, both species possess a small laryngeal opening. As a result of this unique anatomy, visualization of the airway often requires the endoscope to be directly in front of the glottis (see **Fig. 11**). The author has had success intubating both species using a semirigid endoscope with 2.0 to 2.5 mm Cole or uncuffed Murphy endotracheal tubes and with endotracheal tubes constructed from an 8 F red rubber urinary catheter (see **Fig. 4**).[38]

Hedgehog/Sugar Glider

The hedgehog (*Atelerix albiventris*) and sugar glider (*Petaurus breviceps*) can be intubated with a 1.5 mm small exotic straight silicone endotracheal tube or one constructed from other materials. Using the 2.7 mm 30° rigid or the 1.9 mm semirigid scope requires side-by-side intubation. With a 1.0 mm semirigid fiber optic endoscope, however, these species can be intubated successfully using the over-the-endoscope method.

Rats and Other Small Mammals

The author has had repeated success intubating a gray squirrel using a 1.0 mm semirigid fiberscope and a 1.5 mm straight endotracheal tube using the over-the-endoscope technique. This method can be applied to rats and other mammals of similar size. Intubation of mammals smaller than the rat may require the side-by-side technique using either the 1.0 mm small exotic straight silicone endotracheal tube or tubes constructed from intravenous or urinary catheters.[6,34,35]

CONFIRMING PROPER POSITION

Various clinical signs and technical aids are described to verify tracheal intubation.[40–42] These include patient response to intubation (ie, cough), auscultation of the thorax, condensation seen within the tube or on metal placed at the end of the tube, detecting air movement at the end of the tube, listening at the tube opening, and watching the non-rebreathing bag. Additional methods of confirming proper placement include end-tidal capnography,[43,44] tracheal transillumination, chest radiographs, suction of air, and endoscopy (**Fig. 15**).[40,41,45] The use of multiple methods to confirm intubation is recommended.[42] Note that chest compression and positive pressure ventilation are not reliable tests for proper intubation, because air going into and out of the stomach can mimic true chest excursions. Endotracheal tubes should be measured before insertion, and both lung fields should be ausculted after intubation to ensure that the tip of the tube has not passed beyond the bifurcation and into a single bronchus (**Fig. 16**).

Viewing the tube passing between the cords during intubation, and viewing the tracheal rings or the bifurcation endoscopically are the only foolproof methods of confirming proper endotracheal tube placement.[41] Endoscopic intubation allows the intubator an indirect view of the glottis as the endotracheal tube is passed. Further, with over-the-endoscope intubation, the tracheal rings and bifurcation can be seen once the tube is properly placed, which is considered the gold standard for confirming proper placement (see **Fig. 14**).[41]

COMPLICATIONS

Repeated attempts at intubation may prolong anesthesia and injure the glottis. Laryngeal edema, spasm, or perforation may result. Intubation should not be attempted for more than a few minutes, and should be discontinued if there is evidence of trauma. (see **Fig. 14**) Tracheal stenosis has been reported as a result of endotracheal intubation in rabbits and ferrets.[46,47] Scraping the mucosal lining of the trachea has been shown to cause tracheal stenosis in the rabbit.[48] Minimizing trauma to the tracheal lining should avoid this. Patients need to be observed closely while they are intubated. Because of the design of some endotracheal tubes (ie, Cole style), it is easy for accidental extubation to occur with manipulation of the head and neck. Endotracheal intubation significantly increases resistance to airflow through the trachea.[49] As

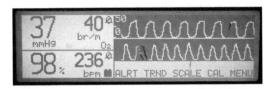

Fig. 15. End tidal capnography and pulse oximetry monitor read-out of a properly intubated rabbit. The rabbit has a ventilation rate of 40 beats per min, with an ETCO$_2$ reading of 37 mm Hg. The pulse is 236 with an partial saturation of oxygen of 98%. (*Courtesy of* Stephen J. Divers, Athens, GA.)

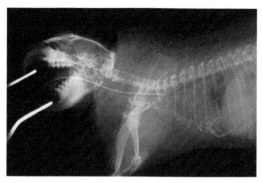

Fig. 16. Excessively deep intubation (shown here in a prairie dog) can be prevented by premeasuring the endotracheal tube before intubation and ensuring proper position with an endoscope afterwards. (*Courtesy of* Dan H. Johnson, DVM, Raleigh, NC.)

endotracheal tube size decreases, airway resistance increases by the inverse of the caliber reduction ratio raised to the fifth power (see **Table 2**). Small endotracheal tubes readily kink and are easily obstructed by mucus and secretions. Due to small patient size, most tubes used for small exotic mammals are uncuffed, and patients are not completely protected from aspiration. If the endotracheal tube gets bitten or the adapter becomes dislodged, aspiration of the endotracheal tube (or portion thereof) can occur. Inadequate ventilation may occur if the endotracheal tube is inadvertently placed too deeply, into a bronchus. Passage of an endotracheal tube can introduce food or fecal mater into the lower airway. Hospital-acquired infection secondary to endoscopic intubation has been reported in people.[27]

DISCUSSION

Endotracheal intubation during general anesthesia is the standard of care for most companion animals, because it offers many advantages over the use of a face mask alone. Intubation makes mechanical ventilation possible; permits the use of a capnograph, apnea alarm, and other monitoring equipment; and facilitates resuscitation should respiratory arrest occur. An endotracheal tube protects against aspiration of gastrointestinal contents, saliva, and blood, and makes it possible to operate on the face and in the oral cavity. Intubation also permits access to the trachea for diagnostic, therapeutic, and research purposes (**Fig. 17**).

In spite of these benefits, many practitioners routinely maintain general anesthesia using a face mask, especially for obligate nasal breathers such as rabbits, guinea pigs, chinchillas, and prairie dogs. This is partly because these species are unable to or rarely vomit, and partly because intubation of these species is difficult. Until recently, few veterinarians received instruction on the intubation of exotic companion mammals. However, as additional methods are developed and perfected, and instruction on the endotracheal intubation of small mammals becomes more widely available, the practice undoubtedly will be accepted as the standard of care for exotic companion mammals also.

Blind intubation takes practice to perfect, requires a breathing patient to perform, and requires the intubator to use a smaller endotracheal tube than is possible with visualization methods. Direct visualization is inherently difficult because of the unique anatomy and physiology of small mammal patients. Intubation via indirect visualization

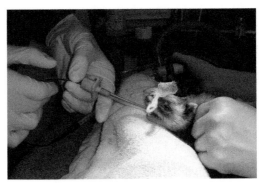

Fig. 17. Tracheal intubation can provide a conduit into the trachea for diagnostic, therapeutic, and experimental purposes. Here, a tracheal wash is performed on a ferret via the endotracheal tube. (*Courtesy of* Dan H. Johnson, DVM, Raleigh, North Carolina.)

reduces anatomic concerns by providing the operator a clear view of the glottis as the endotracheal tube is passed. With all methods of intubation (including side-by-side endoscopic intubation), however, proper placement of the tube must be confirmed. Over-the-endoscope intubation is superior to all other methods in this respect; as the tube is placed into the tracheal lumen, tracheal rings can be seen, confirming that the tube has been properly inserted. With few exceptions, visual methods of intubation require two people to perform. Over-the-endoscope intubation simplifies the intubation procedure by requiring only one. The intubator's eyes, light source, and endotracheal tube are all in one place, so they move in unison.

SUMMARY

Endotracheal intubation has advantages over the use of a face mask for maintaining inhalant anesthesia. Birds, reptiles, and most mammals are intubated routinely, particularly for long anesthetic procedures. Rabbits, guinea pigs, chinchillas and many other small exotic mammals are not, however, because intubation is more difficult to perform. Using a face mask for these species solely on the basis that they are unable to regurgitate ignores the numerous other benefits of airway control.

Although intubation generally improves anesthesia safety, it creates the potential for several new problems. Endotracheal tube obstruction, bronchial intubation, and inadvertent extubation can be avoided as long as practitioners are aware of these complications and monitor patients closely. As long as endotracheal intubation can be performed quickly and safely, exotic companion mammals should receive the same standard of care as other patients.

With the aid of an endoscope, intubation of many small exotic mammals can be accomplished safely and efficiently. The over-the-endoscope technique is the author's preferred method for intubating these animals. The procedure enables intubation to be performed by a single person with relative ease. Like other endoscopic procedures, however, endoscopic intubation of mammals takes practice to perfect.

REFERENCES

1. Davies A, Dallak M, Moores C. Oral endotracheal intubation of rabbits. Lab Anim 1996;30:182–3.

2. Nambiar MP, Gordon RK, Moran TS, et al. A simple method for accurate endotracheal placement of an intubation tube in guinea pigs to assess lung injury following chemical exposure. Toxicol Mech Methods 2007;17(7):385–92.

3. Cantwell SL. Ferret, rabbit, and rodent anesthesia. Vet Clin North Am Exot Anim Pract 2001;4(1):169–91.

4. Heard DJ. Anesthesia, analgesia, and sedation of small mammals. In: Quesenberry K, Carpenter J, editors. Ferrets, rabbits, and rodents: clinical medicine and surgery. 2nd edition. St Louis (MO): WB Saunders; 2004. p. 362–5.

5. Briscoe JA, Syring R. Techniques for emergency airway and vascular access in special species. Sem Avian Exotic Pet Med 2004;13(3):119–25.

6. Lennox AM, Capello V. Tracheal intubation in exotic companion mammals. J Exot Pet Med 2008;17(3):221–7.

7. Freeman MJ, Bailey SP, Hodesson S. Premedication, tracheal intubation, and methoxyflurane anesthesia in the rabbit. Lab Anim 1972;22(4):576–80.

8. Alexander DJ, Clark GC. A simple method of oral endotracheal intubation in rabbits (Oryctolagus cuniculus). Lab Anim Sci 1980;30:871–3.

9. Conlon KC, Corbally MT, Bading JR, et al. Atraumatic endotracheal intubation in small rabbits. Lab Anim Sci 1990;40:221–2.

10. Kruger J, Zeller W, Schottmann E. A simplified procedure for endotracheal intubation in rabbits. Lab Anim 1994;28:176–7.

11. Jaffe RA, Free MJ. A simple endotracheal intubation technic for inhalation anesthesia of the rat. Lab Anim Sci 1973;23(2):266–9.

12. Bertolet RD, Hughes HC. Endotracheal intubation: an easy way to establish a patent airway in rabbits. Lab Anim Sci 1980;30(2):227–30.

13. Haberstroh J, Clancy D, Bönnebrink M, et al. The orotracheal intubation over a retrograde translaryngeal guide in the rabbit. Kleintierpraxis 1993;38(3): 179–80, 182.

14. Davis NL, Malinin TI. Rabbit intubation and halothane anesthesia. Lab Anim Sci 1974;24(4):617–21.

15. Schuyt CH, Leene W. An improved method of tracheal intubation in the rabbit. Lab Anim Sci 1977;27:690–3.

16. Gilroy A. Endotracheal intubation of rabbits and rodents. J Am Vet Med Assoc 1981;183:1295.

17. Hawkins MG, Graham JE. Emergency and critical care of rodents. Vet Clin North Am Exot Anim Pract 2007;10(2):508–10.

18. Turner MA, Thomas P, Sheridan DJ. An improved method for direct laryngeal intubation in the guinea pig. Lab Anim 1992;26:25–6.

19. Kramer K, Grimbergen JA, van Iperen DJ, et al. Oral endotracheal intubation of guinea pigs. Lab Anim 1998;32:162–4.

20. Medd RK, Heywood R. A technique for intubation and repeated short-duration anesthesia in the rat. Lab Anim 1970;4:75–8.

21. Hernandez-Divers SJ, Murray J. Small mammal endoscopy. In: Quesenberry K, Carpenter J, editors. Ferrets, rabbits, and rodents: clinical medicine and surgery. 2nd edition. St Louis (MO): Saunders; 2004. p. 392–4.

22. Vanderhal AL, Berci G, Simmins CF, et al. A videolaryngoscopy technique for the intubation of the newborn: preliminary report. Pediatrics 2009;124(2): 339–46.

23. Weiss M. Video-intuboscopy: a new aid to routine and difficult tracheal intubation. Br J Anaesth 1998;80:525–7.

24. Roark GL. Use of a fiberoptic cystoscope to facilitate intubation in a difficult airway. Trop Doct 2006;36(2):104–5.

25. Platt-Mills TF, Campagne D, Chinnock B, et al. A comparison of GlideScope video laryngoscopy versus direct laryngoscopy intubation in the emergency department. Acad Emerg Med 2009;16(9):866–71.

26. Maktabi MA, Titler SS, Kadakia S, et al. When fiberoptic intubation fails in patients with unstable craniovertebral junctions. Anesth Analg 2009;108(6): 1937–40.

27. Shimono N, Takuma T, Tsuchimochi N, et al. An outbreak of *Pseudomonas aeruginosa* infections following thoracic surgeries occurring via contamination of bronchoscopes and an automatic endoscope reprocessor. J Infect Chemother 2008;14(6):418–23.

28. Boedeker BH, Berg BW, Bernhagen M, et al. Endotracheal intubation in a medical transport helicopter—comparing direct laryngoscopy with the prototype Storz CMAC videolaryngoscope in a simulated difficult intubating position. Stud Health Technol Inform 2009;142:40–2.

29. Costa DL, Lehmann JR, Harold WM, et al. Transoral tracheal intubation of rodents using a fiberoptic laryngoscope. Lab Anim Sci 1986;36(3):256–61.

30. Worthley SG, Roque M, Helft G, et al. Rapid oral endotracheal intubation with a fibre-optic scope in rabbits: a simple and reliable technique. Lab Anim 2000; 34:199–201.

31. Tran HS, Puc MM, Tran JL, et al. A method of endoscopic endotracheal intubation in rabbits. Lab Anim 2001;35:249–52.

32. Vergari A, Polito A, Musumeci M, et al. Video-assisted orotracheal intubation in mice. Lab Anim 2003;37:204–6.

33. Clary EM, O'Halloran EK, de la Fuente SG, et al. Videoendoscopic endotracheal intubation of the rat. Lab Anim 2004;38:158–61.

34. Fuentes JM, Hanly EJ, Bachman SL, et al. Videoendoscopic endotracheal intubation of the rat: a comprehensive rodent model of laparoscopic surgery. J Surg Res 2004;122:240–8.

35. Johnson DH. Over-the-endoscope endotracheal intubation of small exotic mammals. Exotic DVM 2005;7(2):18–23.

36. Lennox AM. Equipment for exotic mammal and reptile diagnostics and surgery. J Exot Pet Med 2006;15(2):98–105.

37. Lichtenberger M. Anesthesia and analgesia for small mammals and birds. Vet Clin North Am Exot Anim Pract 2007;10(2):293–315.

38. Lennox AM. Clinical technique: small exotic companion mammal dentistry—anesthetic considerations. J Exot Pet Med 2008;17(2):102–6.

39. Nixon JM. Breathing pattern in the guinea pig. Lab Anim 1974;8:71–7.

40. Anderson KH. [Methods for ensuring correct tracheal intubation]. Ugeskr Laeger 1991;152(4):267–9 [in Danish].

41. Salem MR. Verification of endotracheal tube position. Anesthesiol Clin North America 2001;19(4):813–39.

42. Rudraraju P, Eisen LA. Confirmation of endotracheal tube position: a narrative review. J Intensive Care Med 2009;24(5):283–92.

43. Swenson J. Clinical technique: use of capnography in small mammal anesthesia. J Exot Pet Med 2008;17(3):175–80.

44. Salthe J, Kristiansen SM, Sollid S, et al. Capnography rapidly confirmed correct endotracheal tube placement during resuscitation of extremely low birth-weight babies (<1000 g). Acta Anaesthesiol Scand 2006;50:1033–6.

45. Cardoso MM, Banner MJ, Melker RJ, et al. Portable devices used to detect endotracheal intubation during emergency situations: a review. Crit Care Med 1998;26(5):957–64.

46. Grint NJ, Sayers IR, Cecchi R, et al. Postanaesthetic tracheal strictures in three rabbits. Lab Anim. 2006;40(3):301–8.
47. Brietzke SE, Mair EA. Laryngeal mask versus endotracheal tube in a ferret model. Ann Otol Rhinol Laryngol 2001;110(9):827–33.
48. Nakagishi Y, Morimoto Y, Fujita M, et al. Rabbit model of airway stenosis induced by scraping of the tracheal mucosa. Laryngoscope 2005;115(6):1087–92.
49. Bock KR, Silver P, Rom M, et al. Reduction in tracheal lumen due to endotracheal intubation and its calculated clinical significance. Chest 2000;118(2):468–73.

Minimally Invasive Surgical Techniques in Bony Fish (*Osteichthyes*)

Mark D. Stetter, DVM, DACZM

KEYWORDS

• Laparoscopy • Fish • Surgery

Aquatic veterinary medicine has seen huge advances over the last decade. In response to the increased value of individual fish, animal welfare concerns, higher standards of care for aquarium fish, and the increased use of fish in research, veterinarians are needed to perform various diagnostic and therapeutic surgical procedures on fish.[1,2] As a taxonomic group, fish represent a tremendous number of different species and huge diversity in size and shape. Relative to domestic animals, very little is known about the diagnosis and treatment of fish. Common veterinary diagnostic tests, such as hematology, auscultation, and palpation are less useful in fish. The fish practitioner often is faced with relatively limited diagnostic options when presented with an ill animal or collection of fish.

Minimally invasive surgery (MIS) provides a great option as a diagnostic tool in fish medicine.[1–4] The ability to directly view individual organs and biopsy tissues is an incredibly valuable tool. MIS in people and other mammals has been shown to have many advantages over traditional surgical procedures.[5,6] Some of these include less postoperative pain, faster healing times, and less chance for infection.[5,6] In fish, MIS has several additional advantages including quicker surgical time and the ability to perform MIS procedures in in situ situations.[1,2] Many fish veterinarians who work with large schools of fish are forced to cull fish for herd health diagnostic purposes. Because laparoscopic surgery allows the clinician to directly image the various organs and collect diagnostic samples, laparoscopy can improve the clinician's diagnostic capabilities and may reduce the need to cull animals for diagnostic sampling.[2]

As the veterinarian is learning laparoscopic techniques in fish, it is recommended that the clinician practice on animals that have died or are being euthanized. This

Department of Animal Health, Disney's Animal Programs, 1200 North Savannah Circle East, Lake Buena Vista, FL 32830, USA
E-mail address: mark.stetter@disney.com

Vet Clin Exot Anim 13 (2010) 291–299
doi:10.1016/j.cvex.2010.01.007
1094-9194/10/$ – see front matter © 2010 Elsevier Inc. All rights reserved.

will allow the clinician to become familiar with both the use of laparoscopic instrumentation and huge variety of anatomy in fish.

The use of a rigid laparoscope in the coelomic cavity of a fish is called coelioscopy.[3,7] Coelioscopy is most commonly used in fish as a diagnostic aid (eg, liver biopsy)[3] or for sex determination[7-12] and less commonly as a therapeutic surgical procedure.[1,2] Standard veterinary laparoscopy equipment can be used easily with fish.[3] The telescope size will be determined by the patient size, but in general, the standard small animal exotic system (2.7 mm × 18 cm, 30° telescope with a 4.8 mm operating sheath) is used commonly with many smaller fish (<8 kg) (**Fig. 1**).[3] In larger fish species, 5 mm and 10 mm telescopes and associated laparoscopic instruments can be used very effectively (**Fig. 2**).[2]

When evaluating coelomic organs, fish usually are placed in dorsal recumbency using a foam wedge to help hold the animal in position (**Fig. 3**). Scales over the incision site are removed, and a scalpel is used to make a stab incision through the skin and underlying muscle tissue. For dorsally compressed species, the incision is made on the ventral midline. A blunt hemostat then is used to enter the coelomic cavity and to enlarge the incision for sheath placement.[1-3,7] In species that are laterally compressed (ie, lie flat from side to side), a general coelomic approach is made via a paramedian incision just cranial to the vent. Depending upon the procedure and the size of the patient, one to three incisions are made for the telescope or instrument ports. From a single incision, the clinician can commonly visualize and sample the following organs: liver, spleen, intestines, stomach, gonads, pericardium, and the serosal surface of the swim bladder (**Figs. 4** and **5**).[2,3,7]

In larger animals, especially if extensive organ manipulation is necessary, other instrument ports commonly are required. In fish that are large enough to accommodate multiple instrument ports, various surgical procedures can be accomplished (**Figs. 6** and **7**). Most trocars and associated instruments come in either 3, 5, or 10 mm sizes. The 3 mm size will be adequate for most procedures in fish.[3]

Insufflation and distension of the coelomic cavity for enhanced organ visualization can be accomplished via traditional CO_2 insufflation or by instilling sterile saline into the coelom.[1-3,7] When using CO_2, pressures of 4 to 8 mm Hg usually provide adequate coelomic distension. In species that have a poorly distendable coelomic cavity,

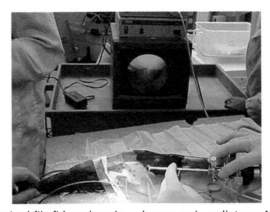

Fig. 1. An anesthetized file fish undergoing a laparoscopic coeliotomy. Note that in highly laterally compressed fish, it is easier to make the incision and enter the coelom from a paramedian incision. (*Courtesy of* Mark D. Stetter, DVM, Diplomate ACZM, Lake Buena Vista, FL.)

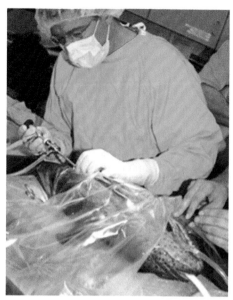

Fig. 2. Laparoscopic coeliotomy in a grouper fish. Note the animal is anesthetized and a water pump is used to flow anesthetic water into the mouth and over the gill arches. The patient is resting on a water-soaked foam pad and has been draped for surgery. (*Courtesy of* Mark D. Stetter, DVM, Diplomate ACZM, Lake Buena Vista, FL.)

pressures in the 8 to 12 mm Hg range may be required. Unlike mammals, which have lungs and a diaphragm, there are no concerns in regards to pulmonary compromise at these higher pressures. High coelomic pressure may have some direct effect on cardiac function, since the coelomic cavity and pericardium are in direct contact; however, this is yet to be determined.[2] It is recommended that as much gas as possible be removed from the coelomic space before closing. Buoyancy problems

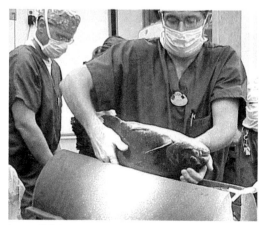

Fig. 3. Anesthetized pacu fish being positioned for surgery. Note that a water-soaked piece of foam has been modified to accommodate this fish in dorsal recumbency. (*Courtesy of* Mark D. Stetter, DVM, Diplomate ACZM, Lake Buena Vista, FL.)

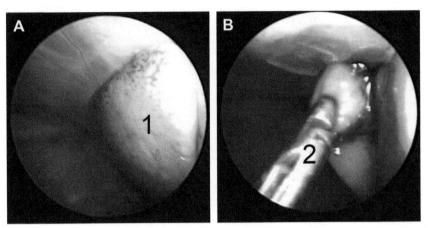

Fig. 4. (A) Laparoscopic view of file fish during exploratory procedure. Note the very pale liver (1). (B) Cup biopsy forceps (2) used to collect a liver sample. Histopathology showed severe hepatic lipidosis. (*Courtesy of* Mark D. Stetter, DVM, Diplomate ACZM, Lake Buena Vista, FL.)

have not been seen commonly after laparoscopic procedures. Saline infusion can be accomplished via an intravenous line attached to the cannula, or a syringe can be attached directly.[3,7] Saline insufflation can be a bit problematic with those animals that have a lot of coelomic fat. Manipulation of organs can cause fat droplet release, which in turn can cloud the saline and obstruct the view, necessitating continued saline flow to maintain visualization. A full-thickness intestinal biopsy can be accomplished laparoscopically by placing a second cannula and inserting a grasping forceps. A loop of bowel is grasped firmly and is pulled up and out of the incision

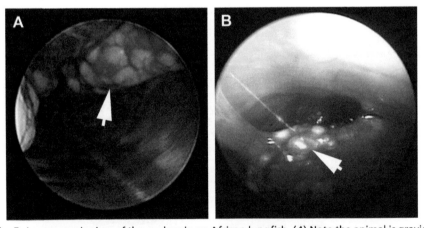

Fig. 5. Laparoscopic view of the coelom in an African lungfish. (A) Note the animal is gravid, and a large number of ova (1) can be seen. Laparoscopy can be used for sex determination in many species of fish. (B) Laparoscopic view of the coelom in a marine angelfish. Note the abnormal white nodular structures of the liver (2). Histopathology of the hepatic biopsy revealed a verminous granulomatous hepatitis. (*Courtesy of* Mark D. Stetter, DVM, Diplomate ACZM, Lake Buena Vista, FL.)

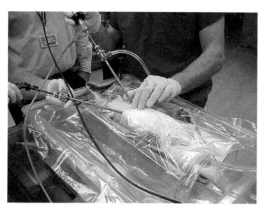

Fig. 6. Laparoscopic exploratory in a sturgeon fish. Note that the large size of this fish allows the use of a 5 mm telescope and associated instruments. The second cannula allows laparoscopic instrument placement for tissue manipulation and biopsy. (*Courtesy of* Mark D. Stetter, DVM, Diplomate ACZM, Lake Buena Vista, FL.)

that has been made for the instrument cannula. This bowel loop now can rest outside the body cavity while the full-thickness intestinal biopsy is performed in the traditional manner. Once the biopsy site is closed, the bowel loop can be pushed back into the coelomic cavity gently.

For procedures that involve either the swim bladder or the kidney, a lateral approach is used commonly (**Fig. 8**). The animal is placed in lateral recumbency, and an incision is made on the lateral body wall, in the caudal half of the swim bladder. Because of the tremendous anatomic variation of the swim bladder among species, it is recommended that a radiograph be taken before the surgery to help confirm the exact location of the swim bladder. A sterile hypodermic needle can be used to help correlate the air bladder's radiographic location with the potential incision site. The needle is placed through the skin at the incision site, and its location relative to the air bladder is confirmed by radiography. Once the incision site is determined, a #11 scalpel blade is used to penetrate the muscular lateral body wall and enter into the swim bladder.[2] In many species, the air bladder is thick and loosely attached to the associated tissues. An aggressive stab incision with the #11 blade allows easier access to the swim bladder and prevents the displacement of the air bladder. Because the swim bladder is only filled with gas, there is minimal risk of tissue damage when it is penetrated. With the laparoscope inside the air bladder, good visualization of the entire internal lining can be accomplished (**Fig. 9**). Evaluation of the swim bladder often requires very little or no insufflation to provide excellent visualization.[2] Please note, unlike coelioscopy in fish, saline should not be used to insufflate or distend the swim bladder. Diagnostic samples can be retrieved easily for cytology, culture, or histopathology. For closure, the swim bladder does not need to be closed separately. One or two sutures through the muscular body wall and the dermis should provide adequate closure.[2]

For renal biopsy, a pair of 4 F laparoscopic scissors can be used to make a small incision through the air bladder wall just over the cranial kidney (dorsocranial aspect of the swim bladder) (**Fig. 10**).[2] Care should be taken to avoid large vessels that may travel along the dorsal midline and are adherent to the air bladder. Biopsy forceps (5 F) are inserted into the instrument channel and fed into the incision site over the kidney.[2] The renal tissue may not be visualized directly, but lies directly dorsal to

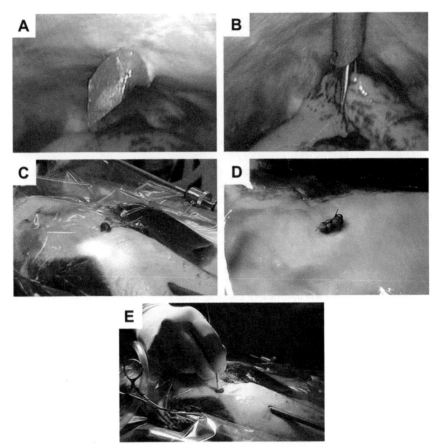

Fig. 7. Sequential images of laparoscopic exploratory with full thickness intestinal biopsy. (*A*) Placement of a second cannula using a sharp trocar after the coelom has been insufflated. (*B*) Grasping of a loop of bowel using a laparoscopic forceps. The loop of bowel is pulled through the body wall incision, while removing the first cannula forceps. (*C*) Loop of intestine has been pulled through the incision and is being prepared for full-thickness biopsy. (*D*) Loop of bowel after a full-thickness intestinal biopsy has been taken and closure is complete. (*E*) Loop of intestinal bowel after biopsy is complete. A wet gauze probe is used to push the loop of bowel back into the coelomic cavity. (*Courtesy of* Mark D. Stetter, DVM, Diplomate ACZM, Lake Buena Vista, FL.)

the swim bladder. Once the biopsy sample has been collected, a surgical gelatin sponge can be placed at the renal biopsy site to help minimize hemorrhage.

Rigid laparoscopy also can be very useful in imaging and sampling the gills and the upper gastrointestinal tract of fish. In those fish species that have small operculum gill filaments (eg, eels, cuttlefish), these can be difficult to see.[1,2] The laparoscope can be used for sample collection by passing the instrument through the opercular slits. Because the esophagus and stomach of most fish species are relatively short and straight, the rigid laparoscope is also useful in evaluating the oral cavity, esophagus, and stomach. Saline can be used to help rinse out the stomach before evaluation. Biopsy forceps can be used to acquire gastric mucosa for direct examination, cultures, or histopathology.

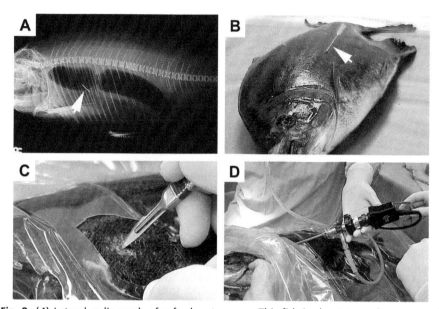

Fig. 8. (*A*) Lateral radiograph of a freshwater pacu. This fish is about to undergo a renal biopsy. Because there is such extensive variation of normal anatomic positions for the swim bladder, a radiograph is used to confirm surgical anatomy. The author prefers to place a hypodermic needle (*arrow*) into the body wall at the proposed incision site and confirm this with a radiograph. (*B*) Anesthetized pacu fish being radiographed, note the hypodermic needle used as a marker (*arrow*). (*C*) Stab incision using a #11 blade into the swim bladder of a pacu fish. The incision should be made after confirmation of swim bladder location with a radiograph. (*D*) Anesthetized pacu fish undergoing renal biopsy taken via laparoscopy. The telescope and associated cannula have been placed through the lateral body wall and into the swim bladder. (*Courtesy of* Mark D. Stetter, DVM, Diplomate ACZM, Lake Buena Vista, FL.)

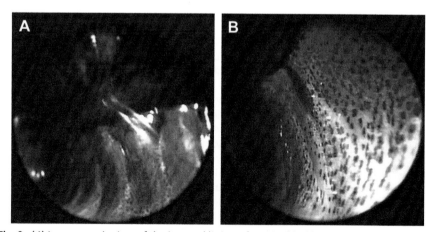

Fig. 9. (*A*) Laparoscopic view of the internal lining of a swim bladder. Note the smooth, clear surface of the swim bladder and the large vessels that run dorsally, just beneath the verte-brae. (*B*) Laparoscopic view of the internal lining of a swim bladder in a freshwater perch. Note the normal areas of pigmentation, which occur in some species of fish. (*Courtesy of* Mark D. Stetter, DVM, Diplomate ACZM, Lake Buena Vista, FL.)

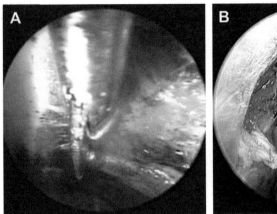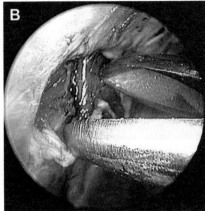

Fig. 10. (*A*) Laparoscopic view of scissors cutting through the dorsal aspect of the swim bladder. Once the incision is complete, biopsy forceps are inserted for liver biopsy. (*B*) Renal biopsy being collected via laparoscopy. Note a small incision has been made through the dorsal aspect of the swim bladder to allow access of the biopsy forceps into the renal tissue. (*Courtesy of* Mark D. Stetter, DVM, Diplomate ACZM, Lake Buena Vista, FL.)

SUMMARY

Rigid laparoscopic surgery can be performed on fish. It is expected that laparoscopy will become a standard technique in veterinary medicine and will provide the zoo and aquarium clinician with a greater variety of diagnostic and therapeutic options. Laparoscopy has been found to be a very effective technique to directly visualize visceral organs and collect tissue samples. Although fish have significantly different anatomy as compared with terrestrial animals, the same laparoscopic principles can be applied successfully to this large and varied group of animals.

REFERENCES

1. Murray MJ. Endoscopy in fish. In: Murray MJ, Schildger B, Taylor M, editors. Endoscopy in birds, reptiles, amphibians, and fish. Tuttlingen (Germany): Endo-Press; 1998. p. 59–75.
2. Stetter MD. Use of rigid laparoscopy in fish. In: Baer CK, editor. Proceedings of the American Association of Zoo Veterinarians. Milwaukee (WI); 2002. p. 339–42.
3. Boone SJ, Hernandez-Divers SJ, Radlinsky M, et al. Comparison between coelioscopy and cocliotomy for liver biopsy in channel catfish (*Ictalurus punctatus*). J Am Vet Med Assoc 2008;233:960–7.
4. Divers SJ, Boone SS, Hoover JJ, et al. Field endoscopy for identifying gender, reproductive stage, and gonadal anomalies in free-ranging sturgeon (*Scaphirhynchus*) from the lower Mississippi River. J Appl Ichthyol 2009;25:68–74.
5. Burrows CF, Heard DJ. Endoscopy in nondomestic species. In: Tams T, editor. Small animal endoscopy. Baltimore (MD): Mosby; 1999. p. 433–46.
6. Cook RA, Stoloff DR. The application of minimally invasive surgery for the diagnosis and treatment of captive wildlife. In: Fowler ME, Miller RE, editors. Zoo and wild animal medicine: current therapy 4. Philadelphia: Saunders Publishing; 1999. p. 30–40.

7. Hernandez-Divers S, Bakal R, Hickson B, et al. Endoscopic sex determination and gonadal manipulation in Gulf of Mexico sturgeon (*Acipenser oxyrinchus desotoi*). J Zoo Wildl Med 2004;35:459–70.
8. Bryan J, Wildhaber M, Papoulias D, et al. Estimation of gonad volume, fecundity, and reproductive stage of shovelnose sturgeon using sonography and endoscopy with application to the endangered pallid sturgeon. J Appl Ichthyol 2007; 23:411–9.
9. Hurvitz A, Jackson K, Degani G, et al. Use of endoscopy for gender and ovarian stage determinations in Russian sturgeon (*Acipenser gueldenstaedtii*) grown in aquaculture. Aquaculture 2007;270:158–66.
10. Moccia RD, Wilkie EJ, Munkittrick KR, et al. The use of fine needle fibre endoscopy in fish for in vivo examination of visceral organs, with special reference to ovarian evaluation. Aquaculture 1984;40:255–9.
11. Ortenberger AL, Jansen ME, Whyte SK. Nonsurgical videolaparoscopy for determination of reproductive status of the Arctic char. Can Vet J 1996;37:96–100.
12. Wildhaber M, Papaoulias D, DeLonay A, et al. Gender identification of shovelnose sturgeon using ultrasonic and endoscopic imagery and the application of the method to the pallid sturgeon. J Fish Biol 2005;67:114–32.

Endoscopy in Sharks

Michael J. Murray, DVM

KEYWORDS

• Endoscopy • Laparoscopy • Elasmobranch • Shark

If one uses mainstream entertainment media as a measuring tool, sharks must be one of the most popular predators on the planet. Couple that with the veritable explosion in the popularity of the public aquarium throughout the world over the past two decades and sharks are commonly encountered in modern society. Newer, more sophisticated life support systems and artificial seawater technology has permitted newer aquaria, and their sharks, to move away from marine coastal areas and into inland population centers. The increased public interest in the aquatic habitat and its inhabitants has been accompanied by an enhanced awareness of the impact that man has upon the fresh and marine waters of the planet. This change in attitude has carried into the captive management of the fish. No longer is the treatment of choice for the fish merely replacement therapy. The same applies to sharks. Diagnostic modalities, including modern endoscopic technologies, are used to aid in the diagnosis, treatment, and prevention of disease in these fish.

Non-veterinarian scientists have long worked with free-ranging shark species. Many of their efforts have been restrained by limitations placed by the size of the shark in hand, the need to accomplish work in field settings, and the anatomic and physiologic constraints associated with invasive procedures. Although still in its infancy, use of minimally invasive technologies are beginning to gain acceptance in a variety of projects involving free-ranging fish.[1]

These changes have placed an increased emphasis on the veterinarian's ability to diagnose and subsequently treat disease, and safely collect a myriad of biology samples, in the shark. At the same time, the availability of high quality rigid endoscopic equipment has increased. Although rigid endoscopy has typically been applied to terrestrial species in the veterinary field, modifications of human-use equipment are easily used in the piscine patient. These fine-diameter, rigid endoscopes permit the veterinarian visualization of a variety of coelomic structures with minimal invasiveness. A sheath system may be added allowing the collection of a variety of targeted biopsy specimens for evaluation, or in animals of adequate size, multiport entries may be used.[2] Rigid endoscopy with its inherent focal, directed illumination with magnification allows the clinician the opportunity to directly visualize coelomic structures and collect diagnostic samples for an etiopathogenic diagnosis, even in species often deemed problematic, such as sharks.

Monterey Bay Aquarium, 886 Cannery Row, Monterey, CA 93940, USA
E-mail address: mmurray@mbayaq.org

Vet Clin Exot Anim 13 (2010) 301–313
doi:10.1016/j.cvex.2010.01.008
1094-9194/10/$ – see front matter © 2010 Elsevier Inc. All rights reserved.

The use of endoscopy in fish is not a novel idea. Although limited, there are some reports of the use of the rigid endoscope as a diagnostic aid in piscine species. Most applications suggest the laparoscope for evaluation of reproductive status in fish. In an early report, a single-puncture technique using a 1.7 mm rigid telescope with a 2.0 mm trocar sleeve is described.[3] In this report, insufflation is accomplished through the injection port associated with the trocar sleeve. Other researchers have described the use of the genital pore as an access point, when the indication for laparoscopy is the determination of reproductive status.[4] A limited description of the use of laparoscopy in the shark has also been published.[5] The information presented here is an attempt to combine the technology employed in human and nondomestic species to several shark species.

EQUIPMENT

Equipment required for endoscopy in sharks is dependent upon severeal factors, including the indication for use, species of shark, size of shark, and the location at which the procedure is to be performed. In general, however, either a rigid pediatric 30-degree Hopkins telescope or a longer, more durable 4 mm, zero-degree Hopkins telescope, depending upon the size of the shark and the target organs, is typically appropriate. Portability of equipment is often of paramount concern, because many procedures are performed tank side or at sea. A combination video screen, camera, image capture device, and light source, such as the Tele Pack (Karl Storz Endoscopy, Goleta, CA) is the preferred system (**Fig. 1**), however, more modern innovations facilitate use of compact, easily transported (and protected from the elements) systems including camera, video monitor, image capture, and light source.

It is possible to employ a modified cystoscope sheath, such as those often used in avian endosurgery (**Fig. 2**); however, some form of peripheral seal is needed to assure that insufflated gas or fluid does not leak around the sheath. The primary advantage of this system, however, is the ability to use a single-entry technique for examination and sample collection. In most cases, an appropriately sized cannula is preferred. The

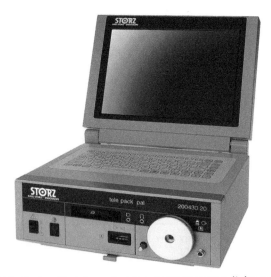

Fig. 1. Portable Tele-Pack with inherent video monitor, xenon light source, camera, and image capture capabilities. (*Courtesy of* Karl Storz GmbH & Co. KG, Tuttlingen, Germany.)

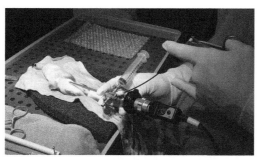

Fig. 2. Use of the traditional avian endoscopy sheath to collect a liver biopsy in a juvenile swell shark (*Cephaloscyllium ventriosum*) using a 12-cc syringe and room air for insufflation. (*Courtesy of* Michael J. Murray, DVM, Monterey, CA.)

Ternamian Endo-Tip cannula with its inherent thread-like exterior permits a more controlled entry into the often restricted spaces within the shark coelomic cavity (**Fig. 3**). Unless one is simply performing an exploratory procedure, cannula use will mandate multiple-entry techniques.

A variety of hand instruments are available for either tissue collection or manipulation. The reader is directed to traditional endosurgical texts for more specific information, as further discussion and description is beyond the scope of this presentation.

INDICATIONS

In general, the indications for endoscopy in sharks mirror those described for other species. Although sharks are sexually dimorphic, endoscopy may be used for reproductive staging or examination of the reproductive tract. A variety of diagnostic specimens, such as tissue biopsies, fine-needle aspirates, microbiological specimens, and parasite removal or identification, are all facilitated endoscopically. As the role of minimally invasive technology has increased in nondiagnostic veterinary science, laparoscopy for the collection of samples for evaluation of contaminants, gene-expression, and so forth is becoming more commonplace. Although not yet statistically validated, it is anticipated that the use of endoscopic methods for the collection of liver biopsies will prove safe and effective in sharks as has been described in other fish species.[6]

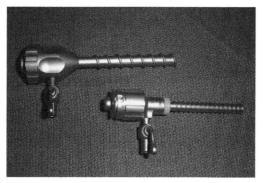

Fig. 3. Ternamian endotip cannula, 6 mm top, 3.9 mm below. (*Courtesy of* Michael J. Murray, DVM, Monterey, CA.)

As a result of the popularity of sharks as exhibit specimens in public aquaria, captive breeding does not keep pace with demand. Therefore, most sharks are wild caught. One study in blue sharks (*Prionace glauca*), revealed that approximately 3% of the blue sharks captured by recreational fishermen had retained fishing hooks from previous capture events.[7] As a result, varying degrees of proliferative peritonitis, hepatitis, and gastritis were identified. Minimally invasive endoscopic techniques may prove appropriate for the management of similar cases in sharks acquired for display in aquariums.

Unlike the traditional teleost fish, gill filaments are tightly affixed to a sheet of muscular and connective tissue, the interbranchial septum (**Fig. 4**).[8] This structure is not accessible through a large opercular opening, but instead through one of several gill slits. As a result, visual examination and subsequent biopsy of the gill is problematic in sharks without the use of endoscopy.

ANESTHESIA

Fish physiologists continue to argue whether or not sharks perceive pain. All agree that the shark is capable of sensing environmental cues, but it is not clear whether noxious stimuli are recognized as such within the central nervous system. That being said, however, veterinarians should probably err on their patients' behalf and administer appropriate forms of anesthesia to preclude pain sensation, assuming there is such a thing in the shark. Regardless of their ability to sense pain, these animals will definitely respond, often violently, to the minimally invasive techniques associated with laparoscopy. The force of the struggling piscine patient is best not unleashed against the delicate nature of the rigid endoscope and associated equipment. Therefore, some consideration for anesthesia is appropriate.

Unfortunately, one size does not fit all. There is variability in the response to chemical agents. Temperature has a great deal of influence on drug response. In most cases, shark temperature and water temperature are equivalent, but some species,

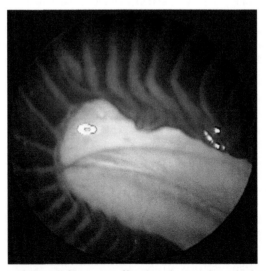

Fig. 4. Arrangement of the gill filaments affixed to the interbranchial septum in the spiny dogfish shark (*Squalus acanthias*). (*Courtesy of* Michael J. Murray, DVM, Monterey, CA.)

such as porbeagle, mako sharks, white sharks, and thresher sharks, are capable of some degree of endothermy making this assumption problematic. Additionally, the influence of hepatic exposure to the drug may modify its affect. Similarly, renal influences may play a role, particularly the theoretical effect of the renal portal system. Unfortunately, one cannot consistently extrapolate the effects of sedatives or anesthetics from mammals to sharks, or even from teleosts to sharks. There may be binding site differences or the activation of these sites may result in an unanticipated, untoward effect. As a result, it is incumbent upon the clinician to extensively research the published scientific literature, gray literature, and most importantly, solicit input from experienced colleagues before using chemical restraint. Specific considerations for pre-immobilization factors and monitoring during the procedure are beyond the scope of this presentation, however, warrant significant emphasis by the clinician.

Tonic Immobility

Many species of shark may be immobilized by positioning them in dorsal recumbency, tonic immobility.[9] Although the shark is typically quite tractable once inverted, there may be significant struggling and excitement during the inversion process. Inverted sharks may require ventilatory support in the form of directed water flow over the gills, and some species should have their tails manually pumped to aid cardiac function. Many minor procedures may be performed under tonic immobility (TI); however, the degree of restraint is highly variable between species and individuals (**Fig. 5**). In field settings, however, TI may be the only immobilization method possible, particularly in large sharks. In such cases, covering the eyes with moistened chamois cloth, combined with well-targeted, rapid procedures and potential use of local anesthesia in the skin are often indicated.

Oxygen Narcosis

Sharks held in water with elevated dissolved oxygen levels (120%–200%) are typically adequately sedated for a variety of minor procedures, often including endoscopy. This effect is variable between species and individuals, and may also vary at differing temperatures. This narcosis effect is most likely the result of a buildup of CO_2 secondary to respiratory depression. Prolonged exposure to elevated CO_2 levels

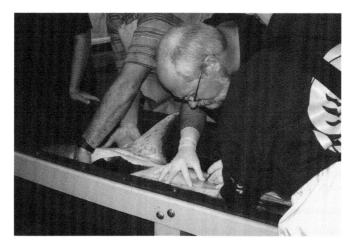

Fig. 5. Laparoscopic approach in a sevengill shark (*Notorynchus cepedianus*) restrained with tonic immobility tank side. (*Courtesy of* Michael J. Murray, DVM, Monterey, CA.)

may result in a severe acidemia. In some cases, there may be significant behavioral changes observed during the recovery period, including aimless swimming, entrapment in tank corners, and failure to avoid obstacles. For that reason, assisted and monitored recovery is recommended.

Tricaine Methane Sulfonate

Tricaine methane sulfonate (MS-222) is a commonly used inhalation anesthetic in a variety of fish species, including sharks. It has also been used at lower doses as a sedative or as a preanesthetic. Induction doses of 50 mg/L followed by a maintenance dose of 10 mg/L have been advocated for sedation during transportation. For anesthesia, most sharks are induced with doses of 80 to 100 mg/L and maintained at levels of 60 to 75 mg/L. The ability to alternate between anesthetic laden and ambient water gives the anesthetist better control over anesthetic depth and duration. In freshwater systems, MS-222 must be buffered. Although this is not so critical in seawater, many advocate buffering in sea water systems with bicarbonate at a ratio of 2:1 bicarb: MS-222. It appears that MS-222 is excreted through the gills and the rate is controlled by cardiac output. In those cases in which output is significantly reduced, recovery may be delayed. Therefore, recovery should be monitored closely.[10]

Injectable Agents

Sedatives or anesthetics may be administered via injection. Intramuscular injections are best given into the muscle of the dorsal saddle. Although some species of shark have red muscle and white muscle, the theoretical differences in drug absorption caused by variation in blood supply have not been well investigated nor clinically appreciated in sharks. The tough skin of the shark mandates use of large needles, 16 to 18 Ga. Additionally, shark skin tends not to self seal, therefore back leakage of injected agents is common. For that reason, directing the needle either cranially or caudally may mitigate some loss of drug. As with any other species, large volumes should be administered in multiple sites to prevent sequestration and abscessation.

Intravenous administration is also possible in the shark. The most commonly used vessels are the caudal vein (ventral tail vein) and the posterior cardinal veins. The caudal vein is located on the midline just ventral to the vertebral column and may be approached either ventrally or laterally. The posterior cardinal vein may be accessed just caudal lateral to the dorsal fin.

Propofol

Slow infusion of propofol (2.5 mg/kg) intravenously has resulted in a surgical plane of anesthesia in spotted bamboo sharks. Induction periods of approximately 5 minutes have been reported with recovery (return of righting reflex) in 60 to 75 minutes. Sharks anesthetized with this protocol remained stable as defined by cardiac and respiratory rates.[11]

Carfentanil/Fentanyl

To date, these opiates have had no effect on sharks, even when administered at massive doses. It is suspected that their failure to respond is related to receptor site differences.[12]

Tiletamine/Zolazepam

This drug combination has been reported to cause hyperexcitability, irritability, and unrestrained biting when administered to sand tiger sharks. It seems doubtful that this combination has much use in shark restraint.

Ketamine/Medetomidine

Initial evaluation of this combination in sharks appears promising. Dosage regimens seem to show a great deal of variability, with some providing surgical anesthesia and others partial sedation. An advantage to this combination appears to be the smooth induction and recovery. Reversal of the alpha-agonist, medetomidine, can be accomplished using atipamezole. It is anticipated that further work on this combination in a wider variety of species will be rewarding.[10]

ANATOMY

As with any surgical procedure, a thorough knowledge of anatomy is critically important for the shark endoscopist. In particular, the ability to understand and predict regional anatomy is paramount when dealing with the typically elongated body form of the shark, which frequently exceeds the working length of endoscopic telescopes and hand instruments. Fortunately, the pertinent gross coelomic anatomy of the shark is consistent between species. As previously described, the anatomy of the gills is significantly different than that encountered in teleost fishes, but again, excepting the number of gill slits, remains consistent in shark species (**Fig. 6**A, B).

As in other fish, the heart is located caudal to the gills within a fluid-filled pericardial space. Generally, this space is visible through a translucent wall at the cranial aspect of the coelom during laparoscopy. In many shark species, the peritoneal cavity has a direct connection to the pericardial cavity via the pericardioperitoneal canal.[13] In the normal shark, this canal is not patent unless the pressure in the pericardial space exceeds that within the peritoneal space. Cardiac stroke volume may then be regulated by movement of fluid from the pericardial space to the peritoneal space during periods of activity. Chronic occlusion of this canal has been shown to result in decreased survival time in horn sharks (*Heterodontus francisci*).[14] The importance and function of this anatomic idiosyncrasy is unclear when peritoneal pressures exceed those in the pericardial space, such as seen during coelomic insufflation. However, its presence and function should be recognized and considered whenever insufflation is necessary.

The most important coelomic structure to the endoscopist is the liver. This organ is typically exceptionally large, often making up nearly 25% of the body weight, is bilobed with a slightly to moderately larger right lobe, and may actually run the entire length of the peritoneal cavity. The high-fat content of the organ serves as an energy source and impacts sharks' buoyancy, as sharks do not have a swim bladder. Endoscopically the liver is typically light brown to yellow in color, as one might expect given the fat content of the structure. The gall bladder is not present in all shark species.

As expected, the J-shaped stomach is located slightly to the left of center; however, its position is often influenced by the quantity of ingesta. The small intestine is short emptying into the morphologically variable spiral colon. Sharks have a discrete pancreas, often closely associated with the spleen or the pylorus. The spleen itself is typically elongated, dark red in color, and may be bilobed. The kidneys are paired, retroperitoneal structures located in the more caudal aspects of the coelom. In the caudal coelom, dorsal to the colon is the fusiform rectal gland, which is intimately involved in osmoregulation.

The reproductive system of the shark is often visualized endoscopically. The male's paired testes are typically noted on either side of the more midline spiral colon. Females may have either single or paired ovaries and oviducts. Unique to some of the sharks is the epigonal organ, a granulo- or hematopoietic organ located in the

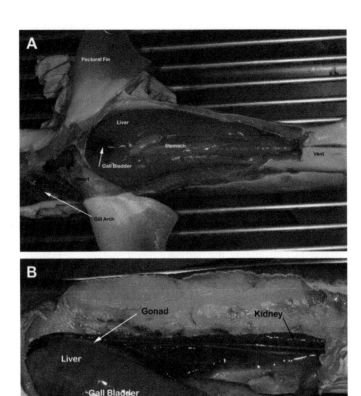

Fig. 6. (A) Dissected, superficial coelomic anatomy in a juvenile scalloped hammerhead shark (*Sphyrna lewini*) in a ventral view. Note how far caudally the liver extends in this specimen. (B) Dissected, superficial coelomic anatomy in a juvenile scalloped hammerhead shark in a lateral view. Note the location of the gall bladder in this species, the retro-peritoneally located kidney, and the small gonad in this juvenile shark. (*Courtesy of* Michael J. Murray, DVM, Monterey, CA.)

gonadal mesentery. The size and appearance of this structure varies between shark species.

One additional anatomic idiosyncrasy of significance to the endoscopist is the presence of the paired abdominal pores located on either side of the cloaca. These structures connect the cloaca, and therefore the environment, with the peritoneal cavity. Their exact function is unclear; however, it is suspected that they have a role in osmoregulation. Their presence may confound efforts to create an adequate visual space via insufflation.

LAPAROSCOPY

As with any other species, laparoscopy should be performed using an aseptic technique. With the shark in dorsal recumbency, insertion points may be gently prepared using a povidone-iodine solution. In most cases, access to the coelomic cavity is gained through a paramedian approach just cranial to the vent. In larger sharks, it may be necessary to move the insertion point further cranially, however, caution to avoid iatrogenic puncture of the large liver must be practiced. By moving the insertion further laterally, access to the kidney is simplified. A sterile, clear drape may be used to isolate the surgical field. As towel clamps are excessively traumatic, the drape may be adhered to the fish by pressing it into a thin bead of gel placed around the incision. The barrier must be substantial enough to keep water out of the incision because the area should be periodically moistened to keep the fish's skin from drying out (**Fig. 7**).

Attempts to visualize viscera without distention of the body cavity are problematic. The tightly packed coelomic cavity leaves little room for instrument manipulation without iatrogenic trauma. If the coelom is distended with saline infused through the injection port of the trocar sleeve, working space is increased, but visualization may becomes difficult as a result of suspension of fat droplets within the instilled saline. Because sharks rely on NaCl, urea, and trimethylamine as major components in plasma osmoregulation, one might question the wisdom of infusing adequate quantities of physiologic saline into the peritoneal cavity of a shark.[15] If one assumes that fluids and electrolytes are absorbed across peritoneal surfaces in sharks as in other species, insufflation with elasmobranch-balanced salt solution[16] may be more appropriate.

Traditional insufflation with carbon dioxide gas is, in the author's experience, the preferred technique. Carbon dioxide is inert, noncombustible, and appears to be well tolerated by the patient. In human and veterinary laparoscopy, carbon dioxide is the insufflation gas of choice.[17] In the shark, as much CO_2 as possible should be removed from the coelom at the end of the laparoscopic procedure. Residual gas appears to have no significant effect on the animal's ability to maintain its position and posture within the water column. In field settings where CO_2 insufflation is not feasible, no side effects with ambient air have been noted to date.

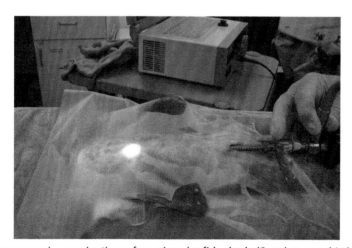

Fig. 7. Laparoscopic examination of a spiny dogfish shark (*Squalus acanthias*). In most species of shark, location of the tip of the endoscope can be identified by the light glow through the body wall. In this case, a 3.9-mm Ternamian cannula has been used to provide access into the coelomic cavity by the endoscope. Insufflation is being provided by the semi-opaque silicone tubing attached to the cannula. (*Courtesy of* Michael J. Murray, DVM, Monterey, CA.)

Use of a Veress needle provides the best insufflation. Following appropriate skin preparation, a 1-mm stab incision is made just through the skin with a #11 scalpel blade. In larger sharks, fine hemostatic forceps may be used to gently dissect partially through the body wall to facilitate a more controlled entry of the Veress needle. The Veress needle is then gently advanced at an angle just off parallel to the skin to enter the coelomic cavity. This increased tunneling, contrary to the perpendicular approach employed in mammalian laparoscopy, facilitates a more water-tight seal after the needle has been removed. Additionally, the body wall cannot be elevated in the mammalian fashion; therefore, a shallower angle decreases the chances of iatrogenic trauma. One may verify entry into the coelomic cavity by the epidural space test. In this test, a drop of saline placed within the hub of the Veress needle will disappear into the lower pressure of the peritoneal space when the body wall is minimally elevated. Once the Veress needle is in place, CO_2 insufflation can occur. In most cases, a peak insufflation pressure of 10 mm Hg is adequate. Excessive pressures may cause visceral prolapse through the rectum.

Once the coelomic cavity has been adequately distended, the telescope may be inserted. If the entry point is to be the same as the point of insertion for the Veress needle, the needle may be removed and a trocar cannula inserted with controlled pressure. If a Ternamian Endo-Tip cannula is used, it may be slowly screwed into place. The telescope may then be introduced into the peritoneal cavity via the cannula. If additional access ports are required, they should be place after the initial entry and visual inspection of the coelom.

For secondary or tertiary access ports, the entry site is prepared as previously described, and a 1- to 2-mm stab incision is made through the skin. A pair of fine mosquito forceps may then be used to bluntly dissect between muscle fibers to approach the coelomic cavity. During the placement of additional cannulae, their entry should be monitored via the telescope already in place. After completion of the laparoscopic procedure, as much CO_2 gas as possible should be milked out of the body cavity. If fluid insufflation is used, the fluid may be allowed to remain within the coelomic cavity, however, for reasons previously discussed, pressures should be allowed to equilibrate before closure.

Following the reduction of insufflations pressures, the surgical wounds should be closed. In smaller sharks, single-layer closure is adequate. In the larger specimens, attempts to oppose the peritoneum and muscle layers followed by the skin are more appropriate. In either case, monofilament polydioxanone (PDS II, Ethicon, Inc, Sommerville, NJ, USA) is the preferred suture.

The laparoscopic approach described provides excellent visualization of a variety of viscera (**Fig. 8**A–I). Although in most cases the liver is the most easily examined organ, gonad, spleen, gastrointestinal tract, peritoneal fat, and idiosyncratic organs, such as the rectal gland and the spiral valve, may also be approached. By advancing the telescope cranially, the pericardial space may be noted. Generally, the heart is observable to beat within this cavity. Changing the position of the fish by rotating it to a more lateral position facilitates observation of the more dorsal structures, such as the kidneys.

ENDOSCOPIC EXAMINATION OF THE GILLS

Even for noninvasive, painless procedures, such as endoscopic examination of the gills, some degree of chemical or physical immobilization of the shark is indicated (**Fig. 9**A–D). Once accomplished, the examination may occur with the animal in dorsal, ventral, or lateral recumbency. Generally, gills are approached through the gill slits,

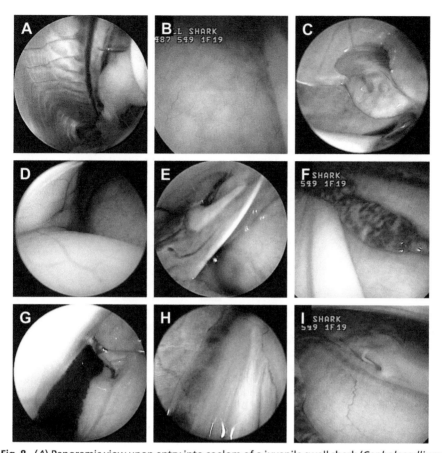

Fig. 8. (*A*) Panoramic view upon entry into coelom of a juvenile swell shark (*Cephaloscyllium ventriosum*). This image has been rotated 180 degrees to place the dorsal midline at approximate 1:00. The pericardial space is visible in the distance, as is the left lobe of the liver. (*B*) Close-up view of the normal liver of the adult sevengill shark (*Notorynchus cepedianus*). The mottled, pale-yellow color is the result of the fat, which serves as an energy depot and aids in buoyancy control, stored within the liver. (*C*) Normal liver and distended gall bladder in a juvenile swell shark. There was no discernible difference between the liver lobes of differing color in this animal. (*D*) Pale-yellow liver, gravid reproductive tract at the bottom of the image, and stomach on the right of the image in a spiny dogfish shark (*Squalus acanthias*). This image is taken with the shark in dorsal recumbency as in **Fig. 7**. (*E*) Liver margin and distended gall bladder in spiny dogfish shark. Note the variability of the gall bladder as compared with that depicted in **Fig. 8C**. (*F*) Reddish-colored spleen in an adult sevengill shark. The mottled surface is not unusual in adult animals. (*G*) Spleen adjacent to the intestine in juvenile swell shark . Compare the surface of the juvenile spleen to that noted in an adult shark, **Fig. 8F**. (*H*) Dorsal-caudal, retroperitoneal kidney in the juvenile swell shark. (*I*) Unidentified parasite in the coelom adjacent to the stomach of an adult sevengill shark. (*Courtesy of* Michael J. Murray, DVM, Monterey, CA.)

however, one may approach via the oral cavity. If the latter approach is used, a rigid speculum should be placed in the oral cavity to protect the instrument and under *no* circumstances should the operator's hands or fingers be placed in the shark's mouth.

Gills may be evaluated either in air or while in water. The quality of the image and subsequently the quality of the examination is enhanced whenever the gills are

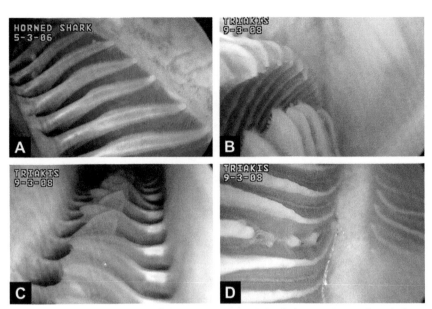

Fig. 9. (*A*) Section of normal gill filament in a horned shark (*Heterodontus francisci*). Note the magnification afforded by the endoscope. (*B*) Gill filaments and individual lamellae in the leopard shark (*Triakis semifasciata*). Examination within an aquatic, rather than aerial environment enhances visualization of individual lamellae. (*C*) Interdigitation of gill filaments within one gill slit in the leopard shark. The somewhat pale appearance of the gill lamellae is indicative of the anemia identified in this specimen. (*D*) Gill damage identified endoscopically in a leopard shark. Although the cause is not confirmed, chronic parasitism is likely. (*Courtesy of* Michael J. Murray, DVM, Monterey, CA.)

allowed to retain the normal architecture seen in water. Therefore, whenever possible, having the head and gills submerged is advantageous. There are occasions when this is not feasible and the clinician must bear in mind the artifact associated with the collapse of the gill filament.

Examinations may be either visual or associated with biopsy. It is recommended that several gill arches be evaluated on both sides and that the examination include the more oral aspect of the structure.

Endoscopy has recently made rapid advancements in human and veterinary medicine. Improvements in optic systems and instrumentation have facilitated the application of endoscopic methods to a variety of species, diagnostic techniques, and surgical procedures. Although the vast majority of the work is done in air breathers, much of it is also applicable to fish, including sharks. Although some idiosyncrasies of form and function exist in this group of fish, they are well suited to endoscopic procedures. As veterinarians gain more insight into the nature of disease of sharks and become more integral in in situ shark research, the utility of this technology will continue to grow.

REFERENCES

1. Divers SJ, Boone SS, Hoover JJ, et al. Field endoscopy for identifying gender, reproductive stage and gonadal anomalies in free-ranging sturgeon (*Scaphirhynchus*) from the lower Mississippi River. J Appl Ichthyol 2009;25(Suppl 2):68–74.

2. Hernandez-Divers SJ. Minimally invasive endosurgery of birds. J Avian Med Surg 2005;19(2):107–20.
3. Moccia RD, Wilkie EJ, Munkittrick KR, et al. The use of fine needle endoscopy in fish for in vivo examination of visceral organs, with special reference to ovarian evaluation. Aquaculture 1984;40:255–9.
4. Ortenburger AI, Jansen ME, Whyte SK. Nonsurgical video laparoscopy for determination of reproductive status of the Arctic char. Can Vet J 1996;37:96–100.
5. Stoskopf MK. Surgery. In: Stoskopf MK, editor. Fish medicine. Philadelphia: WB Saunders; 1993. p. 91–7.
6. Boone SS, Hernandez-Divers SJ, Radlinsky MG. Comparison between coelioscopy and coeliotomy for liver biopsy in channel catfish. JAMA 2008;233(6): 960–7.
7. Borucinska J, Kohler N, Natanson L, et al. Pathology associated with retained fishing hooks in blue sharks, Prionace glauca (L.) with implications for their conservation. J Fish Dis 2002;25(9):515–21.
8. Butler PJ. Respiratory system. In: Hamlett WC, editor. Sharks, skates, and rays. The biology of elasmobranch fish. Baltimore (MD): The John's Hopkins University Press; 1999. p. 174–97.
9. Henningsen AD. Tonic immobility in 12 elasmobranchs: use as an aid in captive husbandry. Zoo Biol 1994;13:325–32.
10. Stamper MA. Immobilization of elasmobranchs. In: Smith M, Warmolts D, Thoney D, et al, editors. Elasmobranch husbandry manual: captive care of sharks, rays, and their relatives. Columbus (OH): Ohio Biological Survey; 2004. p. 281–96.
11. Mitchell MA, Miller SM, Heatley JJ, et al. Clinical and cardiorespiratory effects of propofol in the white spotted bamboo shark (Chiloscyllium plagiosum). In: Proceedings of the 26th annual meeting of the American College of Veterinary Anesthesiologists. New Orleans, October 11–12, 2001. p. 97–112.
12. Stoskopf MK. Shark pharmacology and toxicology. In: Stoskopf MK, editor. Fish medicine. Philadelphia: WB Saunders; 1993. p. 809–16.
13. Tota B. Heart. In: Hamlett WC, editor. Sharks, skates, and rays. The biology of elasmobranch fish. Baltimore (MD): The John's Hopkins University Press; 1999. p. 238–72.
14. Abel DC, Lowell WR, Lipke MA. Elasmobranch pericardial function. 3. The pericardioperitoneal canal in the horn shark (Heterodontus francisci). Fish Physiol Biochem 1994;13(3):263–74.
15. Smith HW. The composition of the body fluids of elasmobranchs. J Biol Chem 1929;81(2):407–19.
16. Andrews JC, Jones RT. A method for the transport of sharks for captivity. J Aquariculture and Aquatic Sciences 1990;5:70–2.
17. Lacy A, Blanch S, Visa J. Alternative gases in laparoscopic surgery. In: Rosenthal RJ, Friedman RL, Phillips EH, editors. The pathophysiology of pneumoperitoneum. New York: Springer-Verlag; 1998. p. 7–17.

Index

Note: Page numbers of article titles are in **boldface** type.

A

Air sacs, avian, vessels examined from during coelioscopy, abdominal air sac, 195, 197–200
        cranial thoracic air sac, 195–196
Airway management, endoscopic approach to. See *Endotracheal intubation.*
Airway resistance, endotracheal intubation impact on, in small mammals, 275, 284–285
Anesthesia, for endoscopy, in avians, 189, 207
        in mammals, 256–257
        in reptiles, 219
        in sharks, 304–307
            carfentanil/fentanyl as, 306
            injectable agents for, 306
            ketamine/medetomidine as, 307
            oxygen narcosis and, 305–306
            propofol as, 306
            tiletamine/zolazepam as, 306
            tonic immobility vs., 305
            tricaine methane sulfonate as, 306
      for endotracheal intubation, of small mammals, 277, 284–286
      for minimally invasive surgery, in bony fish, 292–293
Auscultation, for endotracheal tube position confirmation, in small mammals, 284
Avian endoscopy, diagnostic, **187–202**
        anesthesia for, 189
        biopsy technique for, 196–198
            of kidney, 199
            of liver, 197–199
            of lung, 199–200
            of pancreas, 201
            of spleen, 201
         cloacoscopy as, 191–194
        coelioscopy as, 192
            clavicular approach to, 195, 201
            left approach to, 192, 194–196
                vessels examined from abdominal air sac, 195, 197–200
                vessels examined from cranial thoracic air sac, 195–196
            right approach to, 195, 200
            ventral approach to, 195, 200
        complications of, 201
        contraindications for, 188
        gastroscopy as, 191, 193
        influvioscopy as, 191–192
        instrumentation for, 188

Vet Clin Exot Anim 13 (2010) 315–331
doi:10.1016/S1094-9194(10)00038-1